MEDICAL
INTELLIGENCE
UNIT

VASCULAR GRAFT
MONITORING

Sushil K. Gupta, M.D.

Associate Clinical Professor of Surgery
Harvard Medical School
MetroWest Medical Center
Framingham, MA

R.G. LANDES COMPANY
AUSTIN

MEDICAL INTELLIGENCE UNIT

VASCULAR GRAFT MONITORING

R.G. LANDES COMPANY
Austin / Georgetown

CRC Press is the exclusive worldwide distributor of publications of the Medical Intelligence Unit.
CRC Press, 2000 Corporate Blvd., NW, Boca Raton, FL 33431. Phone: 407/994-0555.

Submitted: February 1993
Published: May 1993

Production Manager: Terry Nelson
Copy Editor: Constance Kerkaporta

Please address all inquiries to the Publisher:
R.G. Landes Company
909 Pine Street
Georgetown, TX 78626
or
P.O. Box 4858
Austin, TX 78765
Phone: 512/ 863 7762
FAX: 512/ 863 0081

ISBN 1-879702-30-4
CATALOG # LN230

CONTRIBUTORS

Dennis F. Bandyk, M.D.
Professor of Surgery
Division of Vascular Surgery
University of South Florida College of
    Medicine
Tampa, FL

Jaap Buth, M.D.
Department of Surgery
Catharina Hospital
Eindhoven, The Netherlands

Richard M. Green, M.D.
Department of Surgery
Chief, Section of Vascular Surgery
University of Rochester School of Medicine
Rochester, NY

Associate Professor of Surgery
University of Rochester School of Medicine
Rochester, NY

Sushil K. Gupta, M.D.
Chief of Surgery
MetroWest Medical Center
Framingham, MA

Associate Clinical Professor of Surgery
Harvard Medical School
Boston, MA

Associate Surgeon
Beth Israel Hospital
Boston, MA

K. Craig Kent, M.D.
Assistant Professor of Surgery
Harvard Medical School
Boston, MA

Attending Surgeon
Division of Vascular Surgery
Beth Israel Hospital
Boston, MA

Raul A. Landa, M.D.
Attending Vascular Surgeon
MetroWest Medical Center
Framingham, MA

Edward Marcaccio, M.D.
Resident
Division of Vascular Surgery
New England Deaconess Hospital
Boston, MA

Arnold Miller, M.D.
MetroWest Medical Center
Natick, MA

Assistant Clinical Professor of Surgery
Harvard Medical School
Boston, MA

Director of Clinical Research
Division of Vascular Surgery
New England Deaconess Hospital
Boston, MA

Luis A. Sanchez, M.D.
Vascular Fellow
Vascular Surgical Services
Montefiore Medical Center
Bronx, NY

Frank J. Veith, M.D.
Chief of Vascular Surgical Services
Montefiore Medical Center
Bronx, NY

Professor of Surgery
Albert Einstein College of Medicine
Bronx, NY

PREFACE

Extensive time and effort are invested by vascular surgeons in implantation of more than 200,000 vascular conduits every year. Despite the great strides made in technical advances and availability of a wide array of choices of graft materials, both natural and synthetic, the essential issue of maintaining graft patency is one that continues to challenge surgeons. Multiple factors influence graft patency including: operative technique, choice of graft material, development of postoperative intimal hyperplasia, patient's coagulation status, and continuation of the atherosclerosis process. Intraoperative and postoperative graft assessment and surveillance have been clearly shown to be important techniques that can be used to detect lesions that threaten graft patency. Correction of lesions leads to prolonged patency.

This book aims to accomplish two goals: the first is to provide surgeons with an overview of techniques with which to monitor grafts so that lesions can be detected early and failure prevented; the second goal is to establish some guidelines for high risk grafts and offer methods of management.

Portions of this book have appeared in journals and published as written proceedings of meetings and symposia.

CONTENTS

1. Graft Failure—Causes and Mechanisms 1
   K. Craig Kent

2. Intraoperative Monitoring of Infrainguinal
   Bypass Grafts 12
   Arnold Miller
   Edward Marcaccio

3. Perioperative Monitoring 34
   Raul A. Landa, Sushil K. Gupta

4. Comparison of Infrainguinal Graft Surveillance
   Techniques 44
   Richard M. Green

5. Duplex Monitoring of the Vascular Graft 55
   Dennis F. Bandyk

6. Surveillance of Lower Extremity Vein Grafts 68
   Jaap Buth

7. Remote Monitoring of Graft Function 79
   Sushil K. Gupta, Frank J. Veith

8. Management of Failing Grafts Detected During
   Surveillance 85
   Luis A. Sanchez, Sushil K. Gupta, Frank J. Veith

9. Epilogue 97
   Sushil K. Gupta

Index 100

CHAPTER 1

GRAFT FAILURE—CAUSES AND MECHANISMS

K. Craig Kent

INTRODUCTION

A successful infrainguinal bypass requires adequate inflow, a nonthrombogenic conduit of sufficient size, and a recipient vessel that adequately perfuses the area of ischemia. Although the quality of the recipient vessel was originally thought to be the most important determinant of graft patency, it is now recognized that excellent results can be achieved with bypasses to diseased tibial vessels and to the small vessels in the foot.[1-4] It has become increasingly clear that the durability of a vascular reconstruction is more closely related to the quality of the conduit that is used.

Five-year patencies approaching 80% can be achieved with greater saphenous vein (GSV) bypass to the popliteal and tibial vessels.[5-7] When the GSV is not available or unusable, other autogenous conduits have been employed, including lessor saphenous, arm or deep femoral vein or endarterectomized native artery.[8-13] These autogenous alternatives are often used only after a previous reconstruction has failed, and it is not surprising that their patency is less than GSV. When used for primary reconstructions, arm and lesser saphenous veins can yield patencies equivalent to GSV.[10,11]

A number of prosthetic conduits have been developed. Polytetrafluoroethylene (PTFE) grafts are used with the greatest frequency. Although reports in the literature vary, prosthetic bypass to the above knee popliteal artery can yield five-year patencies ranging from 42 to 60%.[14-16] Groups achieving high patency rates advocate that above knee femoropopliteal bypass should be performed preferentially with PTFE, even when adequate saphenous vein is available.[16] This "vein sparing" approach allows the saphenous vein to be saved for coronary artery bypass or a later bypass to the tibial vessels. The results of PTFE bypass to the below knee popliteal artery are less impressive, with five-year patencies ranging from 28 to 60%. Prosthetic bypasses to the tibial or pedal vessels rarely remain patent for more than several months.

Initial enthusiasm for umbilical vein grafts stemmed from reports of early graft patencies that were equivalent to greater saphenous vein. Unfortunately, late aneurysmal degeneration is common and often leads to graft failure.[17] Other prosthetic materials, such as dacron, polyurethane and plasma TFE$_{tm}$, have been used clinically or investigated in the laboratory.[18-20] Unfortunately, none of these conduits is able to yield results that are superior to PTFE or equivalent to GSV.

MECHANISMS OF GRAFT FAILURE

Infrainguinal arterial reconstructions are often successful in improving the quality of life in patients with peripheral vascular disease. Unfortunately, not all bypasses remain patent. Under the best of circumstances, early failure occurs with a frequency of at least 5%, and as previously mentioned, at least 20-25% of bypasses will have occluded or required revision by five years. A better understanding of the causes of graft failure might lead to treatments or modifications in technique that will improve both short and long-term patency.

Graft failure that occurs within the first 30 days following surgery is often related to technical misadventure, use of a small or diseased conduit, diminished arterial runoff, or a hypercoagulable state. Graft failures between 1 month and 2 years are often related to hyperplastic lesions that develop within a graft or at its anastomosis with the native artery. Recurrent atherosclerosis accounts for the majority of failures that occur beyond two years. However, these divisions of time are not absolute, and graft failure at any stage can be related to a variety of factors.

EARLY GRAFT FAILURE (30 DAYS)

Early graft failures should occur in less than 5% of infrainguinal reconstructions. However, infrainguinal bypass is technically demanding and a variety of errors can be made.[21]

Choosing the appropriate length for the graft is important, particularly if the bypass crosses the knee or ankle joints. Kinking can occur if the graft is too long. Occasionally, a conduit that is too short will become tethered by fascia or by muscle.

Choosing the proper donor and recipient vessels and the most appropriate sites for anastomoses is equally important. Judgmental errors, such as originating a bypass beyond a hemodynamically significant stenosis or bypassing to a diseased distal vessel, can lead to early graft failure.

Infrainguinal bypass procedures can be tedious and attention to detail is necessary. The actual construction of the anastomosis, particularly a distal anastomosis to a tibial or pedal vessel, requires precise technique using Loupe-magnification and fine suture. Inappropriate handling of the vein or native vessel with forceps, or a misplaced suture, is sufficient to produce graft thrombosis.

Use of a vein that is phlebitic or too small may lead to an unsuccessful bypass. Advocates of the in situ method argue that with this technique, 2-3 mm veins can be successfully used for infrainguinal reconstructions.[22] However, the in situ method has its own technical problems. Vein tributaries that are not ligated may become arteriovenous fistulae, and untransected valves can lead to graft stenosis or occlusion.[21]

The method of vein graft preparation may be an important determinant of early patency. [23, 24] Avoidance of vein graft spasm or over-distention, and perfusion of the vein graft with a physiologic solution may all help to maintain an intact endothelial layer and reduce injury to the media. However, the impact of improved methods of vein graft preparation on early or late graft patency has not been well established.

Although uncommon, hypercoagulable states may contribute to early graft thrombosis. Lupus anticoagulant is an antiphospholipid antibody which interferes with the coagulation pathway. An elevation in the PTT is frequently found, but paradoxically, thrombotic complications are common. How the antibody contributes to thrombosis is unclear. In a retrospective study, Ahn found that 50% of patients with lupus anticoagulant who underwent vascular reconstruction developed graft thrombosis.[25]

Heparin associated thrombocytopenia results from the formation of an autoantibody directed against heparin and the platelet surface.[26] Usually, thrombocytopenia is the only manifestation of this disorder, and discontinuation of heparin will result in a prompt rise in platelet numbers. Occasionally, severe thrombotic complications will develop. This disease process has been noted with increased frequency in patients undergoing hemodialysis, where frequent exposure to heparin is necessary. If heparin associated thrombocytopenia goes unrecognized, the use of heparin during peripheral bypass may lead to graft thrombosis.

Deficiencies in protein S and C have been associated with venous thrombosis, but a relationship between these coagulopathies and arterial thrombosis has not been made. Antithrombin III deficiency may be congenital or acquired and this disorder has been associated with graft thrombosis.[27] Several other hematologic abnormalities can produce a prothrombotic state, including excessive platelet reactivity and diminished levels of plasminogen.[28]

In a recent prospective study, Donaldson[29] screened 158 patients undergoing infrainguinal vascular reconstruction for laboratory evidence of a hypercoagulable state. Early graft thrombosis occurred in 3 of 14 patients with abnormal preoperative tests and only 2 of 123 patients with no abnormalities in their coagulation profile. Of the three patients with coagulopathies who developed graft thrombosis, two were found to have lupus like anticoagulant, and the third was found to have a heparin-induced platelet antibody. Both Eldrup-Jorgensen and Hallett[30,31] found an increased incidence of hypercoagulability in patients under the age of 50; a group of patients in whom the incidence of failed reconstructions is high.

Since the incidence of early graft thrombosis is small and factors other than the state of coagulation contribute to graft failure, it is difficult for studies to accurately reveal the impact of individual coagulation abnormalities on graft patency. Hypercoagulable states are an infrequent cause of early graft thrombosis and a search for these abnormalities should not draw attention away from the technical and judgmental misadventures that often lead to early failure of a vascular reconstruction.

GRAFT FAILURE (ONE MONTH TO TWO YEARS)

INTIMAL HYPERPLASIA (OVERVIEW)

Graft failure that occurs within two years of a vascular reconstruction is often related to intimal hyperplasia.[21,32,33] Histologically, intimal hyperplasia

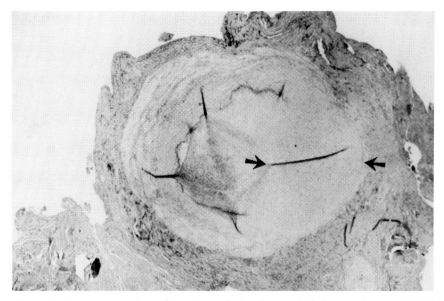

Figure 1. Transverse section of a vein graft that has occluded secondary to intimal hyperplasia. Note the markedly thickened subintimal layer which narrows the lumen of the vein. (between arrows)

is an accumulation of smooth muscle cells (SMC) and matrix within the subendothelial portion of a vessel wall. An initial arterial injury stimulates proliferation of SMC within the media. This is followed by migration of these cells across the internal elastic lamina into the subintimal layer. Continued proliferation of these ectopic SMC, and their deposition of extracellular matrix, leads to vessel wall thickening and luminal narrowing. (Fig. 1) Intimal hyperplasia can develop in endarterectomized vessels, in autogenous vein grafts, at the anastomosis of a prosthetic graft with native artery, or in arteries through which an embolectomy catheter has been passed. Although the exact mode of injury may be different in all of the above circumstances, the end result is a proliferative smooth muscle cell response that can narrow and eventually occlude the lumen.

Although both atherosclerosis and intimal hyperplasia are typified by subintimal proliferation of SMC, there are several notable differences. With atherosclerosis there is an initial migration of lipid-laden macrophages into the subintimal layer. Extensive deposition of lipids eventually leads to the development of a fatty streak which then progresses to an atherosclerotic lesion. As a result, the cholesterol content of atherosclerotic lesions is high compared to intimal hyperplasia.[34] There is also degeneration and necrosis in the central portion of atherosclerotic lesions and eventual calcification. On gross examination, atherosclerotic plaques are irregular and often ulcerated. In contrast, intimal hyperplastic lesions are lacking in lipids. Firm, smooth, glistening white lesions are noted on gross examination. Necrosis and calcification are absent.[35]

Still unknown is the exact nature of the stimulus that activates smooth muscle cell proliferation and migration. Originally, it was thought that the inciting event was a denuding injury to the endothelial layer allowing platelets to attach to collagen in the exposed subendothelial matrix. Release of mitogens, such as platelet-derived growth factor and epidermal growth factor, from aggregating platelets would then stimulate smooth muscle cell proliferation and migration.[34,36]

Recent evidence suggests that platelets may not be the only cell that can promote intimal hyperplasia. Antibodies that effectively inhibit platelet aggregation do not completely obliterate the hyperplastic response that follows an arterial injury.[37] Also, intimal hyperplasia can occur without endothelial disruption.[38,39] Studies have shown that endothelial cells, macrophages and smooth muscle cells all have the potential to mediate this hyperplastic response.

Endothelial cells produce platelet-derived growth factor, fibroblast growth factor, as well as cytokines including interleukin-1 and interleukin-6, all of which are mitogenic for smooth muscle cells.[40] Smooth muscle cells also produce these same mitogens and may, through an autocrine effect, promote their own growth and migration.[41,42]

Unfortunately, the precise stimulus that leads to intimal hyperplasia has not yet been elucidated and may differ with the method of arterial injury. A large number of smooth muscle cell mitogens exists and a variety of cells produce each of these mitogens. An understanding of the exact pathophysiology of intimal hyperplasia will need to await more complex investigations using molecular biologic techniques, including in situ hybridization and cell transfection.[43-45]

INTIMAL HYPERPLASIA (VEIN GRAFT)

Autogenous veins, when used for arterial bypass, develop diffuse microscopic thickening of the intimal layer. This process of "arterialization", is thought to be adaptive and allows the vein to withstand the forces of arterial pressure. Unfortunately, this intimal hyperplastic process can progress, either focally or diffusely, and lead to stenosis or occlusion of a vein graft. (Fig. 2)

The reason why intimal hyperplasia affects some patients and not others is unclear. Cardiovascular risk factors, including hyperlipidemia, smoking, diabetes and hypertension, have been shown to increase the likelihood that intimal hyperplasia will develop. Hyperplasia is frequently found at the site of a venous valve in both in-situ and reversed vein grafts. A traumatic injury from a valvulotome or clamping may be the stimulus that leads to a hyperplastic response. Turbulence related to kinking or the angle of anastomosis may be important, as studies have shown that the propensity to develop intimal hyperplasia is greatest in areas of low shear stress.

Intimal hyperplasia is often limited to the proximal or distal anastomoses, but may develop at any location within the vein graft.[46] Szilagyi was the first to systematically study the biological fate of vein grafts by performing serial angiograms on patients who had undergone femoral popliteal or tibial bypass.[47] He described a number of anatomic lesions that led to vein graft stenoses. Fifty-five percent of these lesions were related to fibrosis or intimal thickening which developed most frequently during the first two years following the initial operation.

Mills recently evaluated the causes for graft failure in 222 reversed infrainguinal bypasses.[48] Fifty-three percent of failures were related to stenoses that were intrinsic to the vein graft. The majority of these lesions were

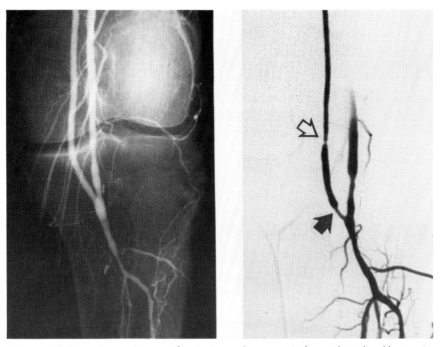

Figure 2. A) Operative angiogram of an in situ saphenous vein femoral popliteal bypass in a 79 year old patient with a nonhealing foot ulcer. B) At the six-month visit, a duplex scan revealed increased velocities in the distal portion of the graft and an angiogram was performed. A focal stenosis within the vein graft is found 3 cm proximal to the popliteal anastomosis (open arrow). A more diffuse hyperplastic response is present just adjacent to the distal anastomosis (closed arrow).

adjacent to or involving the proximal or distal anastomoses (with equal distribution between both anastomoses). Occasionally, either diffuse or focal intimal hyperplasia developed in the mid-portion of the graft. Donaldson identified the cause of failure in 85 in situ saphenous vein grafts.[21] Forty-two graft failures were related to a hyperplastic response. Perianastomotic stenoses developed in 18 grafts; this process was far more common at the distal anastomosis. A stricture of the mid vein graft developed in 14 patients and a focal stenosis in the central portion of the vein was found in 10 grafts.

Intimal hyperplasia might be prevented by modifying a patient's cardio-vascular risk factors or improving surgical techniques so that a traumatic injury to the vein is avoided. Pharmacologic inhibition of smooth muscle proliferation has been successful in animals, but not in humans.[49-51] For the present, intimal hyperplasia remains a relentless and unavoidable cause of failure of autogenous vein grafts.

INTIMAL HYPERPLASIA (PROSTHETIC GRAFTS)

Prosthetic grafts, when placed into the arterial circulation in humans, do not develop a complete endothelial lining. Endothelial cells from the adjacent native vessel migrate only short distances (usually less than 1 cm) into the proximal and distal ends of the prosthetic graft. The remaining graft lumen becomes lined with a "pseudointima" which is composed of fibrin, collagen and several absorbed proteins.

Because the pseudointima is more thrombogenic than an endothelialized autogenous conduit, there is an increased potential for a prosthetic graft to thrombose.[52] This increased potential for graft thrombosis is greatest immediately after implantation, but persists for the life of the graft.

Prosthetic graft failure is not always the result of primary thrombosis, and stenotic lesions related to intimal hyperplasia can develop in the native vessel adjacent to an anastomosis.[53,54] This process occurs far more frequently at the distal anastomosis. (Fig. 3) One possible reason for this propensity is that chronic platelet aggregation occurring in the mid-portion of the prosthetic graft leads to the release of smooth muscle cell mitogens which bathe the distal anastomosis. A hyperplastic response then ensues.

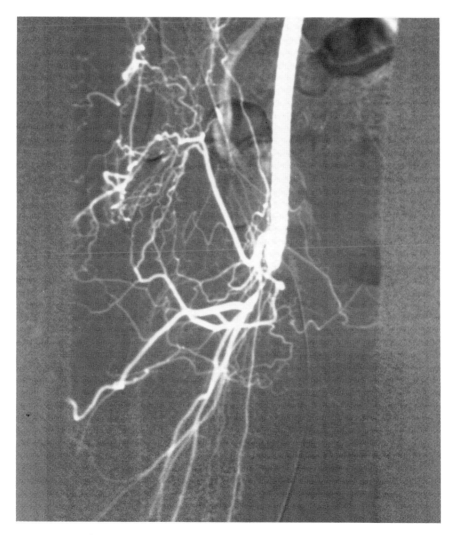

Figure 3. Intimal hyperplasia has developed at the anastomosis of this Dacron aortofemoral graft with the profunda femoris artery. At the time of patch angioplasty, a smooth, glistening, white plaque was found.

LATE GRAFT FAILURE (TWO YEARS)

Progression of atherosclerotic disease is the most common cause of late graft failure. Although atherosclerotic lesions may develop in both the inflow or outflow vessels, the latter is far more common.[21]   The occurrence of significant atherosclerotic disease in the vessels beyond the bypass may be in part related to an initially inappropriate decision at the time of the original bypass regarding the location for the distal anastomosis.

Although late graft failure is often ascribed to progression of atherosclerosis in the inflow or outflow vessels, intrinsic graft lesions are also found. Intrinsic graft lesions discovered beyond two years begin to assume histologic features that are characteristic of atherosclerosis. Szilagyi found atherosclerotic lesions intrinsic to vein grafts as the cause of stenosis in 24% of the diseased grafts.[47] Reifsnyder recently studied 72 autogenous vein grafts using duplex scan (graft age ranging from 4 to 21 years).[54] Fifty-seven percent of grafts were found to harbor abnormalities. Diffuse wall plaque with a less than 50% stenosis was frequently present. Focal stenoses greater than 50% were present in 11/72 graft segments.

Aneurysmal dilatation of vein grafts is a late event noted by both Szilagyi and Reifsnyder.[47,54] However, aneurysms rarely reach a size that is significant enough to produce graft thrombosis. Reifsnyder found that late aneurysms developed in 5 of 7 grafts that had required thrombectomy in the distant past, suggesting that an injury to the vein graft wall at the time of thrombectomy may lead to late aneurysm formation.[54]

MISCELLANEOUS CAUSES OF VEIN GRAFT FAILURE

Sepsis and hypotension are more remote causes of vein graft failure which can occur at any interval following the original bypass. The incidence of limb loss when infrainguinal reconstructions become infected is 50%, although this varies with the type of conduit that has been used. Autogenous bypasses are more readily salvaged than prosthetic conduits. Coverage of the infected autogenous graft with a muscular flap can often prevent graft rupture and thrombosis. With rare exception, infected prosthetic grafts must be removed if infection involves the anastomosis.

Although bypasses will occasionally occlude during an episode of profound hypotension or in patients with severe congestive heart failure, usually such an occurrence is related to an underlying graft stenosis that is not significant when the patient is hemodynamically stable.

SUMMARY

Advances in technique have allowed excellent early and late patencies to be achieved for infrainguinal reconstructions, even with bypasses to the pedal vessels. However, despite the best efforts of those most experienced with these techniques, a late graft failure rate of at least 20% persists. A thorough understanding of the causes of graft failure is a necessary prelude to the development of new techniques and methods that will allow the prevention of graft failure in this subset of patients.

REFERENCES

1. Wengerter KR, Yang PM, Veith FJ et al. A twelve year experience with popliteal to distal artery bypass: The significance and management of proximal disease. J Vasc Surg 1992; 15:143-149.
2. Ascer E, Veith F, Gupta S. Bypasses to plantar arteries and other tibial branches an extended approach to limb salvage. J Vasc Surg 1988; 8:434-441.
3. Harris HW, Rapp JH, Reilly LM, Orlando PA, Krupski WC, Goldstone J. Saphenous vein bypass to pedal arteries: An aggressive strategy for foot salvage. Arch Surg 1989; 124:1232-1236.
4. Buchbinder D, Pasch AR, Verta MJ et al. Ankle bypass: Should we go the distance? Am J Surg 1985; 150:216-219.
5. Taylor LM Jr, Edward JM, Phinney EW et al. Reversed vein bypass to infrapopliteal arteries: Modern results are superior to or equivalent to in situ bypass for patency and vein utilization. Ann Surg 1987; 205:90.
6. Fogle MA, Whittemore AD, Couch NP, Mannick JA. A comparison of in situ and reversed saphenous vein grafts for infrainguinal reconstruction. J Vasc Surg 1987; 5:46-52.
7. Kent KC, Donaldson MD, Couch NP, Mannick JA, Whittemore AD. Femoropopliteal reconstruction for claudication: The risk to life and limb. Arch Surg 1988; 123:1196-1198.
8. Kent KC, Whittemore AD, Mannick JA. Short-term and midterm results of an all-autogenous tissue policy for infrainguinal reconstruction. J Vasc Surg 1989; 9:107-114.
9. Schulman ML, Bradhey MR, Yatco R. Superficial femoral-popliteal veins and reversed saphenous veins as primary femoropopliteal bypass grafts: A randomized comparative study. J Vasc Surg 1987; 6:1-10.
10. Leather RP, Shah DP, Chang BB et al. Resurrection of the in situ saphenous vein bypass: 1000 case later. Ann Surg 1988; 208: 435-442.
11. Harris RW, Andros G, Dulawa LB et al. Successful long-term limb salvage using cephalic vein bypass grafts. Ann Surg 1984; 200:785-792.
12. Inahara T, Scott CM. Endarterectomy for segmental occlusive disease of the superficial femoral artery. Arch Surg 1981; 116:1547-1553.
13. Weaver FA, Barlow CR, Edwards WH, Mulherin JL Jr, Jenkins JM. The lesser saphenous vein: Autogenous tissue for lower extremity revascularization. J Vasc Surg 1987; 5:687-692.
14. Veith FJ, Gupta SK, Ascer E et al. Six-year prospective multicenter randomized comparison of autologous saphenous vein and expanded polytetrafluoroethylene grafts in infrainguinal arterial reconstruction. J Vasc Surg 1986; 3:104-114.
15. Whittemore AD, Kent KC, Donaldson MC, Couch NP, Mannick JA. What is the role of polytetrafluoroethylene grafts in infrainguinal reconstruction. J Vasc Surg 1989; 10:299-305.
16. Quinones-Baldrich WJ, Prego M, Ucelay-Gomez R et al. Long-term results of infrainguinal revascularization with polytetrafluoroethylene: A ten-year experience. J Vasc Surg 1992; 16:209-217.
17. Dardik H, Miller N, Dardik A et al. A decade of experience with the glutaraldehyde-tanned human umbilical cord vein graft for revascularization of the lower limb. J Vasc Surg 1988; 7:336-346.
18. Greisler HP, Dennis JW, Schwartz TH, Kiosak JJ, Ellinger J, Kim DU. Plasma polymerized tetrafluoroethylene/polyethylene terephthalate vascular prostheses. Arch Surg 1989; 124: 967-972.
19. Phua SK, Castillo CE, Anderson JM, Hiltner A. Biodegradation of a polyure-

thane in vitro. J Biomed Mater Res 1987; 21:231-246.

20. Yashar JJ, Thompson R, Bernard RJ et al. Dacron versus vein for femoropopliteal arterial bypass: Should the saphenous vein be spared? Arch Surg 1981; 116:1037-1040.

21. Donaldson MC, Mannick JA, Whittemore AD. Causes of primary graft failure after in situ saphenous vein bypass grafting. J Vasc Surg 1992; 15(1):113-120.

22. Leather RP, Shah DM, Karmody AM. Infrapopliteal arterial bypass for limb salvage: Increased patency and utilization of the saphenous vein used in situ. Surgery 1981; 90:1000-1008.

23. Abbott WM, Wieland S, Austen WG. Structural changes during preparation of autogenous venous grafts. Surgery 1974; 76:1031-1040.

24. LoGerfo FW, Quist WC, Crawshaw HM, Haudenschild C. An improved technique for preservation of endothelial morphology in vein grafts. Surgery 1981; 90:1015-1024.

25. Ahn SS, Kalunian K, Rosove M, Moore WS. Postoperative thrombotic complications in patients with the lupus anticoagulant: Increased risk after vascular procedures. J Vasc Surg 1988; 7:749-756.

26. Sobel M, Adelman B, Szentpetery S, Hoffman M, Posner MP, Jenvey W. Surgical management of heparin-associated thrombocytopenia. J Vasc Surg 1988; 8:395-401.

27. Flinn WR, McDaniel MD, Yao JST, Fahey VA, Green D. Antithrombin III deficiency as a reflection of dynamic protein metabolism in patients undergoing vascular reconstruction. J Vasc Surg 1984; 1:888-895.

28. Towne JB, Bandyk DF, Hussey CV, Tollack VT. Abnormal plasminogen: A genetically determined cause of hypercoagulability. J Vasc Surg 1984; 1:896-902.

29. Donaldson MC, Weinberg DS, Belkin M, Whittemore AD, Mannick JA. Screening for hypercoagulable states in vascular surgical practice: A preliminary study. J Vasc Surg 1990; 11(6):825-831.

30. Eldrup-Jorgensen J, Flanigan DP, Brace L et al. Hypercoagulable states and lower limb ischemia in young adults. J Vasc Surg 1989; 9:334-341.

31. Hallett JW, Greenwood LH, Robison JG. Lower extremity arterial disease in young adults: A systematic approach to early diagnosis. Ann Surg 1985; 202:647-652.

32. Whittemore AD, Clowes AW, Couch NP et al. Secondary femoropopliteal reconstruction. Ann Surg 1981; 193:35-42.

33. Echave V, Koornick AR, Haimov M et al. Intimal hyperplasia as a complication of the use of the polytetrafluoroethylene graft for femoral-popliteal bypass. Surgery 1979; 86:791-798.

34. Ross R. The pathogenesis of atherosclerosis—An update. N Engl J Med 1986; 314:488-500.

35. Dilley RJ, McGeachie JK, Prendergast FJ. A review of the histologic changes in vein-to-artery grafts, with particular reference to intimal hyperplasia. Arch Surg 1988; 123(6):691-696.

36. Ferns GA, Raines EW, Sprugel KH, Motani AS, Reidy MA, Ross R. Inhibition of neointimal smooth muscle accumulation after angioplasty by an antibody to PDGF. Science 1991; 253:1129-1132.

37. Fingerle J, Johnson R, Clowes AW, Majesky NW, Reidy MA. Role of platelets in smooth muscle cell proliferation and migration after vascular injury in rat carotid artery. Proc Natl Acad Sci USA 1989; 86(21):8412-8416.

38. Reidy MA, Chao SS, Kirkman TR et al. Endothelial regeneration. VI. Chronic

nondenuding injury in baboon vascular grafts. Am J Pathol 1986; 123:432-439.

39. Reidy MA. In vivo proliferation of vascular smooth muscle cells in vessels with intact endothelial cover (abstract). Fed Proc 196; 45:683.
40. DiCorleto PE, Bowen-Pope DF. Cultured endothelial cells produce a platelet-derived growth factor-like protein. Proc Natl Acad Sci USA 1983; 80:1919-1923.
41. Majesky M, Reidy M, Benditt EP, Schwartz S. Expression of platelet-derived growth factor (PDGF) A- and B-chain gene in smooth muscle during repair of arterial injury. J Mol Cell Cardiol 1987; 19(suppl IV):S3.
42. Cercek B, Fishbein MC, Forrester JS, Helfant RH, Fagin JA. Induction of insulin-like growth factor I messenger RNA in rat aorta after balloon denudation. Circ Res 1990; 66:1755-1760.
43. Nabel EG, Plautz G, Boyce FM, Stanley JC, Nabel GJ. Recombinant gene expression in vivo within endothelial cells of the arterial wall. Science 1989; 244:1342-1344.
44. Wilson JM, Birinyi LK, Salomon RN, Libby P, Callow AD, Mulligan RC. Implantation of vascular grafts lined with genetically modified endothelial cells. Science 1989; 244:1344-1346.
45. Zwiebel JA, Freeman SM, Kantoff PW, Cornetta K, Ryan US, Anderson WF. High-level recombinant gene expression in rabbit endothelial cells transduced by retroviral vectors. Science 1989; 243:220-222.
46. Veith FJ, Weiser RK, Gupta SK, Ascer E, Scher LA, Samson RH, WhiteFlores SA, Sprayregen S. Diagnosis and management of failing lower extremity arterial reconstructions prior to graft occlusion. J Cardiovasc Surg 1984; 25(5):381-384.
47. Szilagyi DE, Elliott JP, Hageman JH, Smith RF, Dall'olmo CA. Biologic fate of autogenous vein implants as arterial substitutes: Clinical, angiographic and histopathologic observations in femoro-popliteal operations for atherosclerosis. Ann Surg 1973; 178(3):232-246.
48. Mills JL, Fujitani RM, Taylor SM. The Etiology and anatomic distribution of lesions causing reversed vein graft failure: A five-year prospective study. Program for the Society of Vascular Surgery, 46th Annual Meeting, June 8-9, 1992, Chicago, IL., Page 64.
49. Clowes AW, Clowes MM. Kinetics of cellular proliferation after arterial injury. IV. Heparin inhibits rat smooth muscle mitogenesis and migration. Circ Res 1986;58:839-845.
50. Powel JS, Clozel JP, Muller RKM et al. Inhibitors of angiotensin-converting enzyme prevent myointimal proliferation after vascular injury. Science 1989; 245: 186-188.
51. Clowes AW, Reidy MA. Prevention of stenosis after vascular reconstruction: Pharmacologic control of intimal hyperplasia—A Review. J Vasc Surg 1991; 13 (6):885-891.
52. Esquivel CO, Bjork CG, Begentz SE et al. Reduced thrombogenic characteristics of expanded polytetrafluorethyene and polyurethane arterial grafts after heparin bonding. Surgery 1984; 95:102-107.
53. Clowes AW, Kirkman LTR, Clowes MM. Mechanisms of arterial graft failure: Chronic endothelial and smooth muscle cell proliferation in healing polytetrafluorethylene prostheses. J Vasc Surg 1986; 3:877-884.
54. Reifsnyder R, Towne JB, Seabrook GR et al. Biology of long-term autogenous vein grafts—A dynamic evolution. Program for the Society of Vascular Surgery, 46th Annual Meeting, Chicago IL, June 8-9, 1992.

CHAPTER 2

INTRAOPERATIVE MONITORING OF INFRAINGUINAL BYPASS GRAFTS

Arnold Miller
Edward Marcaccio

INTRODUCTION

Since the introduction of infrainguinal bypass grafting in the management of occlusive peripheral vascular disease in the 1950s, there have been dramatic advances both in the refinement of surgical technique and the ability of surgeons to perform more distal revascularization procedures. Graft patency and durability associated with significant improvement in limb salvage has resulted in a dramatic reduction in major primary amputations in patients with advanced occlusive peripheral vascular disease.[1,2] Despite intensive investigation and availability of numerous varieties of small diameter synthetic and biologic prosthetic grafts, none of these conduits have approached the long-term patency of "normal" quality and well prepared autologous vein graft. Autologous vein graft remains the optimal material for the more distal infrainguinal bypass grafts.

Although infrainguinal bypass grafting is generally successful, there remains a significant failure rate within the first month. Failure within the first month is often attributed to operative or technical errors, insufficient "runoff" in the distal vasculature or intrinsic defects within the conduit.

Extensive research effort has been directed toward the development of simple and accurate monitoring techniques to detect correctable defects and improve early graft patency. With the more widespread use of in situ and nonreversed vein bypass techniques and their unique technical demands and the more frequent use of autologous vein other than the saphenous vein, this research has assumed even greater significance.

Clinical assessment of operative technical success is not sufficiently reliable to be used as the sole criterion. While a return of pulse distal to a completed bypass graft is comforting, a palpable pulse does not necessarily equate with increased blood flow. Many popliteal and tibial reconstructions remain patent and the threatened limbs salvaged despite distal arterial disease which precludes return of a palpable foot pulse. Assessment of foot perfusion on the basis of skin temperature and capillary refill time is too variable to be of prognostic value. Foot perfusion is dependent on multiple factors, including anesthetic agents used, intravascular fluid volume status, local vasomotor tone, and the existing collateral circulation.

Useful intraoperative graft assessment must provide surgeons with reliable, objective data with which to evaluate the success of the reconstructive procedure. The ideal intraoperative graft monitoring study must be sufficiently sensitive to detect even minor technical flaws which may contribute to early graft failure, yet, at the same time, possess the specificity to avoid unnecessary postreconstruction interventions. The ideal monitoring technique should be *diagnostic*, to identify and localize such technical errors which contribute to graft failure in order to allow their immediate correction as well as *prognostic*, to determine which grafts are more likely to fail at some time in the future.

Graft monitoring techniques may be indirect, or physiologic assessments, which evaluate the hemodynamic consequences of the procedure or direct, anatomic techniques, which define the technical details of the graft conduit and anastomoses. In this chapter we will briefly review some of the more successful intraoperative "physiological" methods. In addition, we will describe our experience with routine intraoperative angioscopy, and compare it to the intraoperative completion angiogram as direct "anatomic" techniques for preparation of vein conduit and the routine monitoring of autologous vein infrainguinal bypass grafts.

INDIRECT (PHYSIOLOGIC) INTRAOPERATIVE INFRAINGUINAL GRAFT MONITORING

Systematic examination of the efficacy of physiologic measurements to detect technical errors and predict graft outcome began in the late 1950s with a report by Creech et al[3] describing the use of digital plethysmography. Griffin et al in 1971[4] reported on monitoring 19 femoropopliteal bypass grafts with strain gauge plethysmography. They showed no early graft failures in grafts with normal studies. These findings stimulated interest in developing technology. Refinements in plethysmographic equipment resulted in the modern pulse volume recorder[5] a device familiar to most surgeons in the evaluation of the ischemic extremity. O'Donnell et al[6] described direct injection of a pulsed saline solution into the distal artery intraoperatively to monitor femoropopliteal bypass grafts. A baseline pulse volume recording was obtained by using a supramalleolar plethysmographic cuff. This pulse volume was compared to a recording obtained by injecting saline via the open proximal graft end after completion of the distal anastomosis. A final study was obtained with normal flow through the completed graft. Intraoperative angiography to try to identify a technical abnormality was performed when no improvement in the PVR tracing over the baseline study was found. Cumbersome equipment, as well as significant variability associated with injection rates, improper cuff application and changes in vasomotor tone in the early postoperative extremity lead to early abandonment of this technique. Similar variability with poor correlation of outcome[7] was found with application of plethysmography to monitor more proximal reconstructions.

Plethysmography and segmental pressure analysis[8] with a standard blood pressure cuff at the ankle and signal detection by continuous wave Doppler[9,10] have similar problems of variability and subjective interpretation. Use of the audible signals of the continuous wave Doppler, although reassuring to the clinical surgeon, remains qualitative with poor reproducibility and specificity.

Early enthusiasm for intraoperative flow and waveform measurements using the electromagnetic flowmeter (EMF) during intraoperative monitoring of infrainguinal bypass grafting[11-14] soon dissipated as problems of reproducibility were appreciated. Variable measurements with standard deviations of up to 40% can be induced by alteration in probe application to the vessel. Furthermore, the influence of vessel wall characteristics and poor conductivity with ePTFE limits its clinical applicability. Perhaps the most problematic finding was that normal or even high flow rates could occur despite minor technical errors. There also was a lack of specificity in predicting graft failure based on absolute flow rates. While graft flow rates in the 70-100 ml/min range were considered to predict minimal acceptable flow rates, grafts with flow rates as low as 15 ml/min have been shown to have prolonged patency, particularly if constructed with autologous vein. The addition of flow rate measurements enhanced with papaverine injections have not improved the reliability of this technique in predicting patency of infrainguinal bypass grafts.[15-17]

Techniques to measure the "runoff" circulation and thus predict patency were investigated when it became apparent that direct graft flow measurements were poor predictors of technical deficits and graft patency. Stirnemann et al[14] described a direct technique to assess "outflow" volume capacity by a constant pressure saline perfusion over a one-minute time interval. Evaluation of 100 consecutive infrainguinal bypass graft patients undergoing surgery for limb salvage showed that no graft with an outflow capacity of more than 100 ml/min occluded. However, reliable "absolute" threshold criteria were too variable to be of value for routine clinical use.

Similar problems were encountered by Ascer et al[18,19] in determining outflow resistance with a more sophisticated controlled outflow injection technique, coupled with direct pressure transduction and computer assisted resistance calculation. Although they were able to show a higher incidence of graft failure with a higher outflow resistance, the resistance measurement could not identify those grafts which remained patent at least sufficiently long to permit foot lesions to heal and remain healed after graft closure. Furthermore, this method did not identify grafts that failed due to technical defects in the graft or in the proximal inflow vessels, even where the outflow resistance was normal or low.

Velocity waveform analysis using pulsed Doppler ultrasound with spectral analysis together with the B-mode ultrasound (Duplex ultrasound discussed in detail in Chapter 4) is a noninvasive intraoperative monitoring technique that allows discrimination between technical defects and poor graft outflow problems.[20-23] Intraoperative use of pulsed Doppler spectral analysis can identify flow disturbances produced by lesions unassociated with a pressure gradient or reduction in flow volume and may have some predictive value in the determination of graft patency. A major drawback to its routine use in the operating room is the cumbersome equipment, and a somewhat large scanning head that makes it awkward to adequately examine the graft anastomoses[24] particularly in the deeper vessels in the popliteal fossa or the leg. A skilled operator is required for rapid data acquisition and interpretation. To obtain accurate information of flow patterns, the pulsed Doppler sample volume must be placed in the center of the flow stream. Major velocity gradients may be present near the arterial wall. Additionally, low specificity of the flow disturbance data generated and sensitivity of the technique in detecting minor abnormalities which are not reflective of the operative technical errors mandate concurrent anatomic evaluation. This may be accomplished through either angiography or angioscopy prior to attempted revision[25] to avoid unnecessary intervention.

Transcutaneous oxygen tension (TcPO$_2$) determination has been utilized recently as an indirect method of intraoperative graft monitoring. This method was introduced as a definitive technique to predict wound and potential amputation site healing and met with variable success. The intraoperative use of TcPO$_2$ in predicting success of a bypass graft relies on positive responses noticed immediately after completion of the reconstruction. A rise in perfusion index[26] or rise of TcPO$_2$ > 15 torr at 10 minutes[27] have been reported to show a good predictive value of sustained graft patency. Although a simple and relatively easy technique, TcPO$_2$ monitoring suffers from a lack of reproducibility due to its dependence on other hemodynamic factors and measuring difficulties. This method does not allow discrimination between technical flaws in the bypass graft and inadequate distal runoff. Therefore, it cannot identify nor localize conduit or anastomotic errors amenable to intraoperative correction without adjunctive anatomic evaluation.

DIRECT (ANATOMIC) INTRAOPERATIVE INFRAINGUINAL GRAFT MONITORING

Direct techniques in routine clinical use for intraoperative monitoring of infrainguinal bypass grafts are the completion angiogram and intraoperative angioscopy. Routine completion intraoperative angiography[28-32] has been advocated as the method of choice for monitoring infrainguinal bypass surgery since its introduction nearly two decades ago. Most reported studies of completion angiography during bypass surgery are retrospective or anecdotal but the angiogram is still generally regarded as the "gold standard" for monitoring these bypass grafts. Although highly specific, the intraoperative angiogram has only moderate sensitivity in the detection of technical imperfections or native vessel abnormalities that may cause graft failure.[24,33-34]

Intraoperative angioscopy provides direct, in vivo, three-dimensional visualization of the interior of the graft, anastomoses and native vessels. It has been shown to be a safe, effective alternative or adjunct to the intraoperative angiogram.[34-42] Angioscopy has many advantages over the angiogram. Not only is it a useful technique for monitoring the bypass surgery for technical errors and their immediate correction, but angioscopy facilitates vein conduit preparation by allowing selection of optimum vein segments in a diseased vein or ensuring complete valvulotomy in the in situ and nonreversed vein. Angioscopy has delineated "new" previously unappreciated findings that may cause graft failure and stimulates novel ideas for the design and development of new and useful therapeutic intraluminal instrumentation and devices, which may effect changes in current surgical techniques for infrainguinal bypass grafting. [43-45]

TECHNIQUE OF INTRAOPERATIVE ANGIOGRAM

The intraoperative angiogram is usually performed at the completion of the bypass procedure after release of the clamps and resumption of blood flow. The extent of the procedure varies considerably in clinical practice. Some advocate the routine visualization of both anastomoses, the entire graft and the runoff vasculature.[30] Others emphasize the need to delineate the entire vein graft in order to assess completeness of valvulotomy and detection of arterio-venous connections when the in situ technique is used.[46] Most frequently, however, an angiogram is used to evaluate the technical proficiency of the distal anastomosis, continuity and extent of the "runoff" vasculature.

In order to visualize both anastomoses, injection of contrast material is made in the proximal artery, above the proximal anastomosis.[30] Generally, a 19-gauge, butterfly needle is connected to tubing with a 3-way stopcock and a 30 ml syringe with heparinized saline or contrast material (Renograffin 30 or 60). Our own preference is to visualize the proximal anastomosis only if there is a specific problem. During vein preparation a deliberate effort is made to leave a sufficient length of ligated tributary at the proximal end of the graft which can easily be intubated with a Mark's or Titus needle for the angiogram without risk of injury to the vein graft. With use of synthetic material or absence of a suitable tributary, the needle is inserted directly into the graft. Inflow occlusion either of the proximal vessels or the graft proximal to the injection site is useful to ensure complete filling of the graft and runoff vasculature with minimal dilution of the contrast material. Between 15 and 30 ml of contrast material is injected with minimal delay in exposure, as is necessary in the preoperative angiogram. An X-ray cassette is placed directly beneath the region of interest and the lower limb or foot is angled appropriately to display the graft and the lateral profile of the distal anastomosis.

TECHNIQUE AND EQUIPMENT FOR INTRAOPERATIVE ANGIOSCOPY

Intraoperative angioscopy is performed with angioscopes varying in external diameter from 0.8-3.0 mm (Olympus Corporation, Lake Success, NY). The operating room set-up and equipment is shown in Figure 1. Essential equipment includes a CCD chip video-camera, VCR, high resolution video-monitor, video-character generator, microphone, light source and a dedicated irrigation pump. All angioscopic studies are recorded on video tape including the comments of the surgeon and the angioscopist. This enhances interpretation of the intraoperative findings when the study is reviewed.

Our techniques, methods and results of intraoperative angioscopy performed during infrainguinal revascularization have been previously reported.[41-42, 47-48] The technique, like all endoscopy requires skill, knowledge and a great deal of practice. The unique problem of vascular endoscopy is that blood is opaque to all spectra of light so that for consistent high quality angioscopic visualization, the blood needs to be completely displaced from the visual field and replaced with a clear saline solution. Unlike angiography, where a sufficient concentration of contrast media mixing with the blood allows high quality angiograms, in angioscopy, the intraluminal blood must be totally replaced and a clear column of fluid established. A small volume of red cells causes

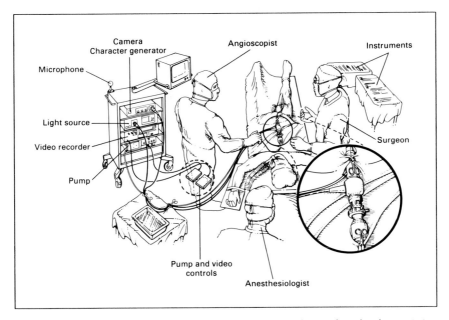

Figure 1. Standard angiography set-up in the operating room. (Reproduced with permission Miller A, Jepson S[47])

blurring of the visual field and the image appears to be "out of focus". The presence of blood makes meaningful visualization impossible.[49]

To achieve complete replacement of the blood with a clear saline fluid column, certain requirements need to be met. All antegrade blood flow, both from the main inflow vessel and the collaterals needs to be halted. Any blood flowing in the same direction as the irrigation fluid will join the irrigation fluid and a clear fluid column will never be established. At surgery this usually entails proximal clamp occlusion of the native arteries or graft. A bolus of fluid, injected at a high flow rate and large volume, is necessary to clear all the blood. The more rapidly the column of clear fluid can be established, the less total fluid will be needed for the angioscopic study.[49] Once the clear column of fluid is established it can be maintained by irrigating at a much lower flow rate and smaller volume, providing this is above the collateral and "backbleeding" pressure. This prolongs the time visualization is possible during angioscopy and minimizes the total volume of irrigation fluid used.

A dedicated irrigation pump for angioscopy[49] was developed together with the Olympus Corporation (Angiopump®). This peristaltic pump is designed to provide flow rates between 10 ml/min and 400 ml/min and to generate a maximum pressure of 2,000 mm Hg at the pump head. The pump provides for the selection of two independent flow rates, a high flow rate or "bolus" and a low flow rate or "maintenance". These flow rate settings are variable, independent of each other and may be adjusted either prior to or during the procedure. Adequate pump settings for most infrainguinal bypasses are approximately 300 ml/min for the "bolus" and approximately 80 ml/min for the "maintenance" flow rates. (Table 1) These settings should be adjusted, increasing the flow rates with the more proximal grafts and greater collateral flow and run-off bed and decreasing the settings for the more distal

Table 1. Pump settings and volume of irrigation fluid used in completion angioscopy of 95 infrainguinal bypass procedures (Modified with permission from Miller et al[41]).

Procedure	#	Pump Settings, ml/min		Total irrigation fluid Volume, ml (Range)
		High (Range)	Low (Range)	
Femoropopliteal	37			
Above knee	15	315 (250-400)	68 (50-90)	436 (0-1400)
Below knee	22	291 (250-300)	62 (50-85)	478 (150-900)
Femorotibial	38	266 (150-300)	66 (50-85)	518 (100-1000)
Femorodorsalis pedis	11	276 (250-300)	44 (0-80)	439 (100-800)
Popliteodorsalis pedis	7	243 (150-285)	75 (50-100)	250 (50-500)
Popliteoposterior tibial	2	248 (220-275)	63 (50-75)	267 (150-450)
Total	95	***	***	398 (0-1400)

bypasses.[41] The flow rate is controlled remotely with a double action foot pedal, allowing switching back and forth, from "bolus" to "maintenance", so that after the column of clear fluid is established it may be maintained at all times in the vessel under examination.

A serious concern is that the rapid infusion of fluid under pressure into a relatively restricted outflow tract, could result in excessively high intra-arterial pressures which would damage the intimal lining or deeper layers of the arterial wall, even to the extent of complete rupture. This does not appear to occur. Both our experimental data[49] and clinical findings[41-42,48] have clearly demonstrated that provided the vessel under infusion is not totally occluded or the infusion is stopped as soon as clearing of the visual field occurs, irrigation at these high flow rates does not appear to cause "clinical" significant injury. Direct measurements of the intraluminal pressure in vein grafts during angioscopy (Fig. 2) have shown that during most of the angioscopy procedure the pressures remained within the physiological range.[50]

The most critical limitation to angioscopy is the volume of irrigation fluid that can safely be infused into a particular patient. In our experience (Table 2), the average volume of fluid routinely required for irrigation with the dedicated irrigation pump to consistently achieve good quality and complete studies is approximately 500 ml (range 50-1500 ml). If the patient is carefully monitored hemodynamically, such volumes have not proven to be a problem. In a prospective, randomized trial comparing intraoperative angiography and angioscopy for the monitoring of vein bypass grafts, no significant difference was demonstrated.[50] We compared the total intraoperative fluid volume used, the incidence of therapeutic maneuvers to treat fluid overload intraoperatively (diuretics or nitroglycerin) or the incidence of cardiac morbidity and mortality, either intraoperatively or in the immediate postoperative period.

Table 2. Size of angioscope and mean volume of irrigation fluid

Procedure	#	0.8 mmOD	1.4 mmOD	2.2 mmOD	2.8 mmOD	3.0 mmOD	mean fluid volume (range ml)
Femoropopliteal							
Above knee	28	-	16	11	1	-	458 (64-1412)
Below knee	53	2	29	20	1	1	410 (51-904)
Femorotibial	163	10	130	20	1	1	419 (50-1098)
Femoropedal	57	8	41	8	-	-	433 (77-1160)
Popliteodistal	54	7	45	2	-	-	218 (37-625)
TOTAL	355	27	261	61	3	3	397 (37-1412)

Reproduced with permission from Miller et al[49]

For each angioscopic application, a standard method of angioscopic examination is utilized according to the operative procedure and the nature of the region of interest. In the in-situ or the nonreversed vein bypass, angioscopy is performed during vein preparation and again at the completion of the procedure in lieu of or as an adjunct to the intraoperative angiogram.

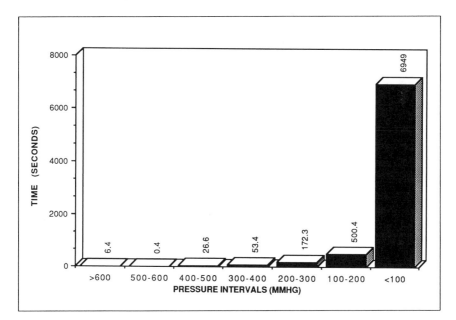

Figure 2. Intraluminal graft pressures generated during 24 completion angioscopies for infrainguinal bypass grafts and their duration are shown in this graph. (Reproduced with permission from Kwolek et al[50])

In the reversed vein graft or the synthetic graft, angioscopy is performed upon completion of the distal anastomosis after the clamps have been removed and the blood flow re-established, either prior to or after tunneling the graft. Where the information is of critical importance, such as the site of an anastomosis or assessment of the adequacy of the distal artery, angioscopy is performed prior to the revascularization procedure.

For routine bypass surgery, only the distal artery, the distal anastomosis and the graft are routinely examined as a completion monitoring procedure. Retrograde or upstream angioscopy to examine the proximal artery and anastomosis is performed only in selected cases where inflow problems are suspected.

The largest angioscope relative to the smallest vessel necessary to be intubated is always chosen. This avoids the danger of inducing spasm in the vein graft or the native artery and also allows passage through the diseased and stenotic artery thus allowing a complete study. For infrainguinal bypass grafting we have found angioscopes of approximately 1.4 mm external diameter to be the most useful. (Table 2) Irrigation is almost always performed through a separate irrigation catheter or needle inserted collateral to the angioscope (Fig. 3) or through a large irrigation sheath with a proximal hemostatic valve, coaxial with the angioscope. Flow rates achieved through the angioscopes with built-in irrigation channels, even with the dedicated angioscopy pump, are inadequate for most successful angioscopic studies during infrainguinal bypass.[49] Furthermore, angioscopes with larger irrigation channels and higher flow rates are almost always too large and rigid to be inserted through the distal anastomosis and into the distal artery, particularly in bypasses distal to the popliteal arteries.

To ensure completeness of the angioscopy study, it is important to visualize the entire lumen of the vessels under study. This may be achieved by using a steerable angioscope or by manipulating a nonsteerable angioscope. Steerable angioscopes not only enhance the quality of the angioscopic study but are much easier to manipulate intraluminally than the standard nonsteerable angioscope. The nonsteerable angioscopes may be "steered" by rolling or torqueing the angioscope between the plantar surfaces of the thumb and index finger so that the entire vessel circumference can be visualized. Direct external manipulation on the distal end of the angioscope through the vessel wall is another method of ensuring full visualization of the entire lumen and in particular, the anastomosis. Coordinating these manipulations is best achieved by watching the images produced on the monitor and making adjustments accordingly, and not by attempting to directly position the angioscope tip within the anastomosis or lumen of the vessel or graft by force. These techniques significantly enhance the value of the studies and aid the surgeon in gathering the relevant information.

COMMENT

Perhaps the most important advantage of the intraoperative angiogram is that the operative technique is well established and it is readily available in most operating rooms. Its main shortcoming, however, apart from the occasional allergy and anaphylaxis reaction to the contrast material or induction of acute tubular necrosis, is that the X-ray is a single unidimensional projection that often obscures significant intraluminal pathology or technical errors which could possibly have been detected with a different projection. In addition, the angiogram has an inherent weakness in delineating the details of intraluminal pathology. While significant or complete obstruction to flow is well defined, subtle intraluminal abnormalities, such as mural thrombus, recannalized vein, nonobstructing flaps and intimal injuries or residual competent valves in the in situ vein graft are frequently overlooked. The contrast material surrounds the intraluminal pathology. Depending on the projection, the contrast will display it or hide it from view. Finally, poor mixing of the contrast material with blood or sluggish blood flow, or accidental injection of small volumes of air may manifest as filling defects and be interpreted as abnormalities in the completion angiogram resulting in unnecessary surgical

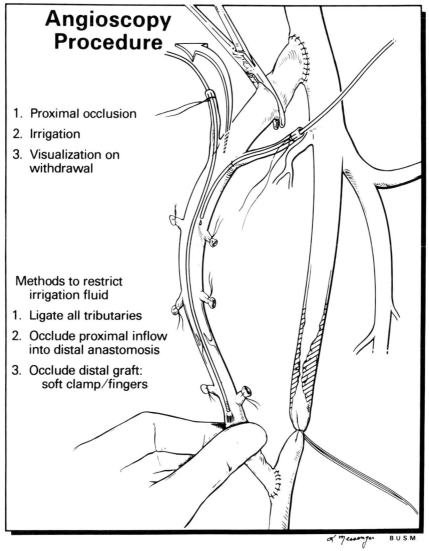

Figure 3. Standard technique of completion angioscopy for infrainguinal bypass grafts. (Reproduced with permission Miller A, Jepsen S [51])

interventions. (Fig. 4) The incidence of false positives has not been well documented but appears to vary between 1-3%.[30] However, in our own series of 122 consecutive intraoperative angiograms, out of 7 abnormal findings, 2 (28.6%) were false positives and resulted in unnecessary interventions.[51]

A review of recent reports of intraoperative angioangiography is instructive. Over the last two decades, there has been a dramatic reduction in the number of technical errors detected when completion intraoperative angiogram is performed routinely. This is true despite extension of the bypass grafts to the tibial and even the pedal vessels. Although synthetic or "biologic" conduits were common in the early studies, even in those studies where autogenous vein was the most frequently used conduit, almost all of the abnormal findings detected were confined to the region of the anastomosis or the artery just distal to the anastomosis. The reported incidence of these findings was between 2%-6%.[28-30]

These findings are in direct contrast to our experience with the routine use of the angioscope during infrainguinal bypass grafting. Most of the abnormal findings requiring intervention were in the vein graft conduit.

Between May 1, 1987 and August 31, 1992, we have performed intraoperative angioscopy during more than 950 revascularization procedures including infrainguinal bypass grafting, thrombectomy or embolectomy, carotid endarterectomy and coronary artery bypass grafting. Our largest experience with angioscopy is for infrainguinal bypass grafting and this experience has previously been extensively reviewed.[41-42,48]

Figure 4. Completion angiogram showing a "filling" defect in the anastomosis of a femoroposterior tibial reversed saphenous vein bypass graft. (Reproduced with permission from Miller et al[45])

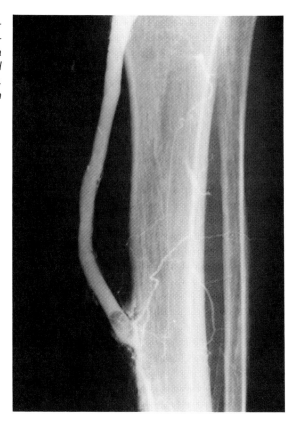

Table 3. 155 clinical or surgical decisions in 355 infrainguinal bypass grafts

A. Graft

(In situ 197, NRV 93, RV 44, PTFE 8, Composite PTFE-Vein 13)

Residual competent valve leaflets	40	(17.3%)*
Unligated tributaries	65	(32/9%)
Graft torsion/inadequate graft tunnelling	2	
Recanalized vein	23	
vein discarded	3	
recannalized segment excised	6	
webs/bands/strands cut	14	
Vein stenosis		
segment excised	2	
venoplasty	1	

B. Anastomosis/Distal Artery

Revision of anastomosis	9
technically inadequate	2
postanastomotic stenosis	4
intimal flap	3
Thrombectomy of distal artery	2
Primary siting of anastomosis	7

C. Miscellaneous

Post-op LMD/heparin for intraluminal platelet thrombus	4

Total	**155**

*angioscopic valve lysis in 57
(Reproduced with permission from Miller et al.[48])

These studies have clearly demonstrated that the routine use of angioscopy as a monitoring procedure during infrainguinal bypass surgery is clinically useful, safe and effective. Table 3 lists the clinical decisions made during a retrospective review of our experience with the first 355 infrainguinal bypass grafts. More than two-thirds of the bypasses were infrageniculate and in more than 96% of the bypasses the graft conduit was autogenous saphenous vein. Intraoperative clinical surgical decisions were made in 155 of the 355 bypasses or 43.6%. Analysis of these decisions show that most of these decisions, (105/155, 67.7%) related to the special technical requirements for use of the grafts in the in situ vein and nonreversed configurations. Nevertheless, 28/155 (18%) findings were related to unsuspected intraluminal vein pathology and occasional technical problems related to the tunneling of the vein graft. Only 18/155 (11.8%) of the bypasses abnormal findings were associated with the anastomosis and distal artery.

We have shown that the standard "blind" technique of valvulotomy with a retrograde valvulotome for the in situ and nonreversed vein is associated with a consistent incidence of residual competent valve leaflets, approximately 20% and 6% respectively, despite a continuous and extensive experience with this "blind" technique. (Fig. 4) In some cases these residual valves may be responsible for graft failure.[23,39,52] We and others have shown that cutting valves under angioscopic direction obviates the problem of residual competent valves[44-45,53-55] and in addition, avoids valvulotome induced injury to the vein.[45] Our technique for angioscopically directed valvulotomy and valvulotome are shown in Figure 5.

Primary intraluminal pathology in veins, either saphenous or arm vein, is a common cause of graft failure. Even complete vein exposure and careful external examination of the vein detects intraluminal pathology in only a small percentage of abnormal veins. The incidence of such pathology in 53 consecutive completion angioscopies in saphenous vein bypass grafts extending from the groin to the ankle or into the foot is shown in Table 4. In arm vein used for infrainguinal bypass grafts, the incidence of intraluminal pathology is much more frequent, between 60-70%.[56-57] This may reflect the problems associated with this unique patient population. Typically, these patients suffer from multiple illnesses, recurrent hospitalizations, and associated repeated phlebotomy and intravenous infusions. Figure 6 shows the distribution of these findings in the veins of the upper extremities noted in in the preparation of 113 consecutive arm vein conduits undergoing infrainguinal reconstruction.

Segmental areas of previous thrombosis and recanalization, (Fig. 7) seen endoscopically as webs, bands or strands are the most prominent pathology. Excision of diseased areas of the vein that are dense and limited in length or cutting the webs or bands under angioscopic direction with the retrograde valvulotome when the lesions are fine or sparse, enables the surgeon to

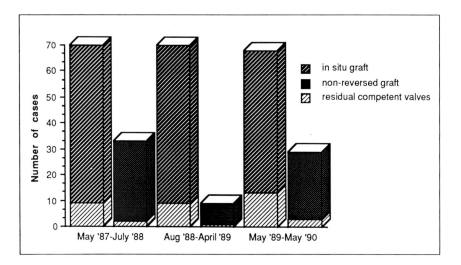

Figure 5. The incidence of retained competent valves following "blind" retrograde vavulotomy in vein graft preparation in the in situ and nonreversed bypass grafts during three arbitrary time periods of data analysis:
a. Between May 1987-July 1988, 12/52 (23%) in situ and 2/31 (6.5%) nonreversed;
b. Between August 1988-April 1989, 9/61 (14.8%) in situ and 1/8 (12.5%) nonreversed and;
c. Between May 1989-May 1990, 13/55* (23.6%) in situ and 3/26* (11.5%) nonreversed.
*the 28 in situ and 27 nonreversed veins prepared by angioscopic directed valvulotomy

Table 4. Endovascular pathology noted in 22 of 53 in infrainguinal saphenous vein bypass grafts extending from the groin to the ankle

N = 53	#	%
Sclerotic or thickened vein segments	11	20.7
Recanalization (webs/bands/strands)	7	13.2
Thickened or sclerotic valves	4	7.5
Organized thrombus (discrete regions)	2	3.8

(Modified with permission from Miller et al.[48])

upgrade the final vein conduit quality. To obtain an adequate length it is often necessary to build a composite vein conduit with multiple segments anastomosed together. Review of 109 consecutive infrainguinal bypasses using only arm vein show that 71 of the veins had intraluminal pathology.[57] Angioscopically directed interventions of these veins allowed "upgrading" of the quality in 64 (90%) of these veins with conduits that were made of composite segments. The early and one-year primary patency of these up-graded conduits was not different from the normal quality arm vein conduits used in the study. If problems with these conduits are undetected at the time of bypass surgery, there is a high incidence of early graft failure.[56] As a result, a reluctance to use arm vein has been prevalent since the initial arm vein experience was reported in the literature. In a small, retrospective, nonrandomized study comparing arm vein bypasses monitored with angioscopy and completion angiogram, we showed a 30-day primary patency of 100% in 27 consecutive arm vein bypasses as compared to only 82% in 57 bypasses where the completion angiogram or continuous wave Doppler was used to monitor the bypass grafts.[56]

These studies have led to a concept of "inferior" vein conduit, which recognizes the importance of vein quality in the durability of the graft. Definition of such vein is made with angioscopic criteria looking at regions of thrombosis and recanalization (webs/bands/strands), sclerotic and stenotic segments or adherent intraluminal thrombus and occasionally on clinical criteria, which includes vein size (<2.5 mm external diameter), external sclerosis or stenosis. Evaluation of the vein with either venography or Duplex ultrasound[58] does not detect such endoluminal pathology unless it involves long segments of the vein or causes significant stenosis.

Although our previous studies[56,57] clearly demonstrated the advantages of vein preparation and monitoring with intraoperative angioscopy in the "inferior" vein, the question remains as to whether angioscopy, with the additional expense of the new instrumentation and learning curve of a new technique, should be instituted routinely as the "ideal" monitoring technique for infrainguinal bypass grafting.

A prospective and randomized study was conducted to determine whether an improvement in the early (<30 day) graft patency could be demonstrated in primary infrainguinal bypass grafts using only saphenous vein as the graft conduit when routine monitoring with intraoperative angioscopy rather than

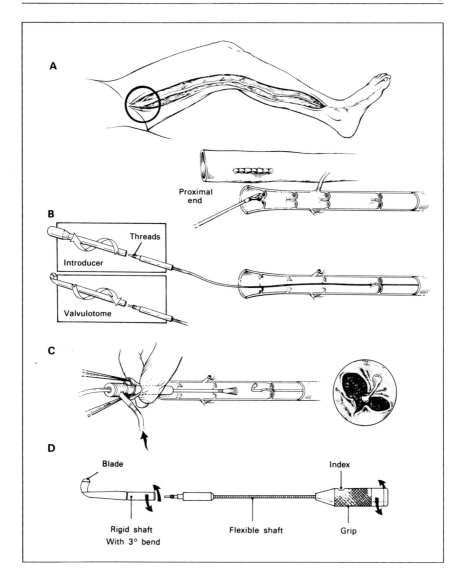

the "gold" standard intraoperative completion angiogram was performed. Although our study demonstrated a trend in favor of the angioscope as the better technique for the routine monitoring of the bypass graft it did not reach statistical significance in the select group studied. (Fig. 8) There were many reasons for this lack of statistical significance, but perhaps the most important was the universal preference by all the participating surgeons in using the angioscope whenever the quality of the vein was in question.[51]

The most striking difference between the two monitoring modalities is illustrated in Table 5 which shows the total number of surgical interventions performed following completion of monitoring studies in 250 randomized bypass grafts, 32 with completion angioscopy and only 7 with completion angiogram (p < 0.0001). Furthermore, most of these interventions were associated with the use of vein conduit, 28 with completion angioscopy and only 1 with completion angiogram (p < 0.0001). The number of interventions in the distal anastomosis and "runoff" artery, was not significantly

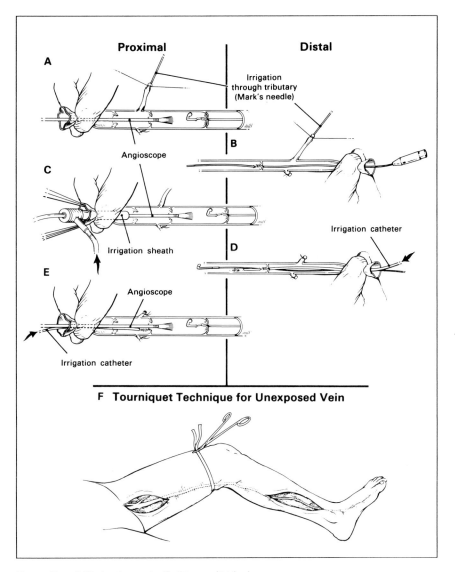

Figure 6i and 6ii. Angioscopically Directed Valvulotomy.

6i—A-D Technique (opposite page): A. The saphenous vein is completely exposed and the tributaries ligated. The patient is heparinized and the vein transected at both ends. The vein is gently distended with papevrine saline solution and the first proximal valve excised with scissors; B. The valvulotome with introducer in place is passed through the vein from the distal end to protrude through the proximal end of the vein. The introducer is replaced with the appropriately sized valvulotome; C. The valvulotome is withdrawn under constant angioscopic direction steering past the tributary orifices and accurately cutting each valve leaflet; D. The valvulotome.

6ii—Alternative methods of irrigation (above): A. Irrigation through a Mark's needle inserted through a tributary at the proximal end of the vein; B. Irrigation through a Mark's needle inserted through a tributary at the distal end of the vein; C. Irrigation sheath (7-9 French) with hemostatic valve allows for passage of angioscope and proximal irrigation; D. Irrigation catheter (16 gauge) for distal irrigation held in place together with valvulotome; E. Collateral irrigation catheter (16 gauge) lying alongside the angioscope for proximal irrigation; F. Tourniquet technique for unexposed vein. The tourniquet is only applied at the time of angioscopically directed valvulotomy. (Reproduced from Miller et al [45])

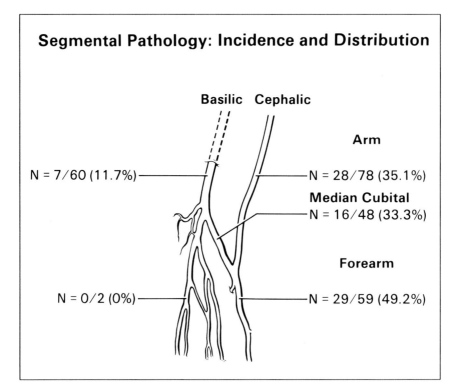

Segmental Pathology: Incidence and Distribution

Basilic Cephalic

Arm

N = 7/60 (11.7%)   N = 28/78 (35.1%)

Median Cubital
N = 16/48 (33.3%)

Forearm

N = 0/2 (0%)   N = 29/59 (49.2%)

Figure 7. The incidence and distribution of the segmental pathology detected with angioscopic preparation and monitoring of 113 arm veins harvested for infrainguinal bypass conduits is illustrated. (Reproduced with permission from Marcaccio et al [57])

different for either monitoring procedure, but unlike the completion angiogram where there were 2 out of 5 false positive studies, there were no false positive findings with completion angioscopy. The two false positive findings following completion angiogram resulted in unnecessary exploration of the distal anastomosis with the early occlusion of one of the bypass grafts.

CONCLUSIONS

Review of the literature[1-2,31-32, 42,46,59] reveals a progressive improvement in patency rates for infrainguinal bypass grafts. This improvement is significant because the population includes severely threatened limbs, very ill and elderly patients, and extension of the grafts more distal in the leg and foot. If the conduit is of good quality and the surgeon proficient in the surgical techniques, good results are possible. In those bypasses where the vein conduit is of good quality, the "runoff" vasculature adequate and the technique proficient, monitoring the bypass surgery for technical or correctable errors does not appear to influence the early graft patency significantly. However, with suboptimal conduits or in patients with borderline "runoff", the role of monitoring the bypass surgery assumes greater significance.

Our studies [41-42,48,51] and those of others [24,34] clearly show that intraoperative angioscopy is the most efficient way to monitor these autogenous vein grafts, the anastomoses and adjacent distal artery for correctable intrinsic

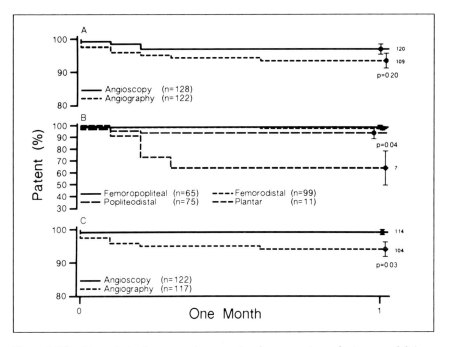

Figure 8. Life table analysis of one month comparing the proportions of primary graft failure. 1. Of the angioscopy and angiogram groups, the difference at one month is not statistically significant (p=0.2). 2. Of the 11 bypasses to the plantar arteries and the remaining 239 bypasses in the study, at one month the difference is statistically significant (p=0.04). 3. Of the angioscopy and angiogram groups with the 11 plantar arteries excluded, the difference at one month is statistically significant (p=0.03). (Reproduced with permission from Miller et al [51])

Table 5. Relevant findings and clinical decisions during the completion monitoring procedures of 250 infrainguinal bypass grafts for "nonintervention" and "intervention"

	Nonintervention (N = 14 bypass grafts)		Intervention (N = 36 bypass grafts)	
	Angioscopy	Angiogram	Angioscopy	Angiogram
Vein conduit	5	1	28	1
Residual competent valve	0	0	9	1
Vein preparation/selection	5	1	6	0
Tributary ligation	0	0	13	0
Anastomosis	8	0	3	5
Distal artery	0	0	1	1
Total	**13**	**1**	**32**	**7**

(Modified with permission from Miller et al.[51])

abnormalities or technical defects. Angioscopy also provides an effective way to ensure an optimally prepared graft conduit. The "anatomic" monitoring of the bypass apparently is more specific and accurate than the "physiological" measurements obtained intraoperatively. The physiological measurements are dependent on too many variables to provide specific information relevant to the bypass under examination. In those bypasses where the "runoff" vasculature has not been clearly delineated in the preoperative angiogram, the addition of an intraoperative angiogram to delineate the outflow tract may provide "anatomic" information to allow optimal placement of grafts and better prediction of outcome. However, for long-term prognostication, the "physiological" rather than the "anatomic" monitoring techniques may provide better information. Physiologic studies performed early in the postoperative period and repeated at frequent intervals may be the most effective way to predict patency of an individual graft [23,25] Furthermore, such postoperative monitoring may allow detection of developing intragraft defects which, if uncorrected, may cause the graft to fail.

REFERENCES

1. Veith FJ, Gupta SK, Wengerter, KR et al. Changing arteriosclerotic disease patterns and management strategies in lower-limb-threatening ischemia. Ann Surg 1991; 212:402-414.
2. LoGerfo W, Gibbons G, Pomposelli F et al. Evolving trends in the management of the diabetic foot. Arch Surg 1992; 127:617-621.
3. Creech O, DeBakey M, Culotta R. Digital blood flow following reconstructive arterial surgery. Arch Surg 1957; 74:5.
4. Griffin L, Wray C, Vaughan B, Moretz W. Detection of vascular occlusions during operation by segmental plethysmography and skin thermometry. Ann Surg 1970; 173:389-397.
5. Darling R, Raines J, Brener B, Austen W. Quantitative segmental pulse volume recorder: A clinical tool. Surg 1972; 72:873-887.
6. O'Donnell T, Raines J, Darling R. Intraoperative monitoring using the pulse volume recorder. Surg, Gyn & Ob 1977; 145:252-254.
7. O'Donnell T, Cossman D, Callow A. Noninvasive intraoperative monitoring: a prospective study comparing Doppler systolic occlusion pressure and segmental plethysmography. Am J Surg 1978; 135:539-546.
8. Williams L, Flanigan D, Schuler J, Lim L. Intraoperative assessment of limb revascularization by Doppler-derived segmental blood pressure measurements. Am J Surg 1982; 144:578-579.
9. Mozersky D, Sumner D, Barnes R, Strandness DJ. Intraoperative use of a sterile ultrasonic flow probe. Surg Gynecol Obstet 1973; 136:279.
10. Barnes R, Garrett W. Intraoperative assessment of arterial reconstruction by Doppler ultrasound. Surg, Gyn & Obstet 1978; 146:896-900.
11. Mannick J, Jackson B. Hemodynamics of arterial surgery in atherosclerotic limbs. Surg 1966; 59:713-720.
12. Barner H, Kaminski D, Codd J, Kaiser G, Willman V. Hemodynamics of autogenous femoropopliteal bypass. Arch Surg 1974; 109:291-293.
13. Bush H, Corey C, Nabseth D. Distal in situ saphenous vein grafts for limb salvage. Am J Surg 1983; 145:542-548.
14. Stirnemann P, Triller J. The fate of femoropopliteal and femorodistal bypass grafts in relation to intraoperative flow measurement: an analysis

of 100 consecutive reconstructions for limb salvage. Surg 1986; 100:38-44.

15. Terry H, Eng C, Tayor G. Quantitation of flow in femoropopliteal grafts. Surg Clin N Am 1974; 54:85-94.

16. Bernhard V. Intraoperative monitoring of femorotibial bypass grafts. Surg Clin N Am 1974; 54:77-83.

17. Dean R, Yao J, Stanton P, Bergan J. Prognostic indicators in femoropopliteal reconstructions. Arch Surg 1975; 110:1287-1293.

18. Ascer E, Veith F, White-Flores S, Morin L, Gupta S, Lesser M. Intraoperative outflow resistance as a predictor of late patency of femoropopliteal and infrapopliteal arterial bypasses. J Vasc Surg 1987; 5:820-827.

19. Ascer E, Veith F, Gupta S. Bypasses to plantar arteries and other tibial branches: an extended approach to limb salvage. J Vasc Surg 1988; 8:434-441.

20. Bandyk D, Zierler R, Thiele B. Detection of technical error during arterial surgery by pulsed Doppler spectral analysis. Arch Surg 1984; 119:421-427.

21. Bandyk D, Cato R, Towne J. A low flow velocity predicts failure of femoropopliteal and femorotibial bypass grafts. Surg 1985; 98:799-809.

22. Bandyk D, Jorgensen R, Towne J. Intraoperative assessment of in situ saphenous vein arterial grafts using pulsed Doppler spectral analysis. Arch Surg 1986; 121:292-299.

23. Bandyk D, Kaebnick H, Stewart G, Towne J. Durability of the in situ saphenous vein arterial bypass: A comparison of primary and secondary patency. J Vasc Surg 1987; 5:256-68.

24. Gilbertson J, Walsh D, Zwolak R et al. A blinded comparison of arteriography, angioscopy, and duplex scanning in the intraoperative evaluation of in situ saphenous vein bypass grafts. J Vasc Surg 1992; 15:121-9.

25. Bandyk D, Kaebnick H, Bergamini T, Moldenhauer P, Towne J. Hemodynamics of in situ saphenous vein arterial bypass. Arch Surg 1988; 123:477-482.

26. Gannon M, Goldman M, Simms M, Hardman J. Transcutaneous oxygen tension monitoring during vascular reconstruction. J Cardiovasc Surg 1986; 27:450-453.

27. Alexander J, Pello M, Spence R, Camishion R. Intraoperative transcutaneous oxygen tension criteria for completion arteriography. Ann Vasc Surg 1990; 4:333-337.

28. Plecha F, Pories W. Intraoperative angiography in the immediate assessment of arterial reconstruction. Arch Surg 1972; 105:902-907.

29. Dardik H, Ibrahim I, Koslow A, Dardik I. Evaluation of intraoperative arteriography as a routine for vascular reconstructions. Surg Gynecol Obstet 1978; 147:853-858.

30. Liebman P, Menzoian J, Mannick J, Lowney B, LoGerfo F. Intraoperative arteriography in femoropopliteal and femorotibial bypass grafts. Arch Surg 1981; 116:1019-1021.

31. Taylor L, Edwards J, Phinney E, Porter J. Reversed vein bypass to infrapopliteal arteries. Ann Surg 1987; 205(1):90-97.

32. Donaldson M, Mannick J, Whittemore A. Causes of primary graft failure after in situ saphenous vein bypass grafting. J Vasc Surg 1992; 15:113-120.

33. Stept L, McCarthy W, Bartlett S et al. Technical defects as a cause of early graft failure after femorodistal bypass. Arch Surg 1987; 122:599-604.

34. Baxter B, Rizzo R, Flinn W et al. A comparative study of intraoperative angioscopy and completion arteriography following femorodistal bypass. Arch Surg 1990; 125:997-1002.

35. Crispin H, Van Baarle A. Intravascular observation and surgery using the flexible fibrescope. Lancet 1973; 1:750-751.

36. Vollmar J, Storz L. Vascular endoscopy. Surg Clin North Am 1974; 54:111-22.

37. Towne J, Bernhard V. Vascular endoscopy: useful tool or interesting toy. Surgery 1977; 82:415-9.

38. Towne J, Bernhard V. Technique of intraoperative endoscopic evaluation of occluded aortofemoral grafts following thrombectomy. Surg Obstet Gynec 1979; 148:87-89.

39. Grundfest W, Litvack F, Glick D et al. Intraoperative decisions based on angioscopy in peripheral vascular surgery. Circulation 1985; 78(suppl I):I-13-I-17.

40. Mehigan J, Olcott C. Videoangioscopy as an alternative to intraoperative arteriography. Amer J Surg 1986; 152:139-145.

41. Miller A, Campbell D, Gibbons G et al. Routine intraoperative angioscopy in lower extremity revascularization. Arch Surg 1989; 124:604-8.

42. Miller A, Stonebridge P, Jepsen S et al. Continued experience with intraoperative angioscopy for monitoring infrainguinal bypass grafting. Surgery 1991; 109:286-93.

43. White R. Technical frontiers for the vascular surgeon: Laser anastomotic welding and angioscopy-assisted intraluminal instrumentation. J Vasc Surg 1987; 5:673-80.

44. Chin A, Fogarty T, ed. Specialized techniques of angioscopic valvulotomy for in situ vein bypass. Chicago: Year Book Medical Publishers, Inc, 1989:76-83. (White G, White R, ed. Angioscopy: vascular and coronary applications.

45. Miller A, Stonebridge P, Tsoukas A et al. Angioscopically directed valvulotomy: a new valvulotome and technique. J Vasc Surg 1991; 13(6):813-821.

46. Leather R, Shah D, Chang B, Kaufman J. Resurrection of the in situ vein bypass: 1000 cases later. Ann Surg 1988; 208:435-442.

47. Miller A, Jepsen S, ed. Angioscopy in arterial surgery. Philadelphia: W.B. Saunders Company, 1990:409 - 416. (Bergan J, Yao J, ed. Techniques in Arterial Surgery

48. Miller A, Stonebridge P, Kwolek C. The role of routine angioscopy for infrainguinal bypass procedures. In: Ahn S, Moore W, eds. Endovascular Surgery. 2nd ed. Philadelphia: W. B. Saunders Co, 1992:

49. Miller A, Lipson W, Isaacsohn J, Schoen F, Lees R. Intraoperative angioscopy: Principles of irrigation and description of a new dedicated irrigation pump. Am Heart J 1989; 118:391-9.

50. Kwolek C, Miller A, Stonebridge P et al. Safety of saline irrigation for angioscopy: results of a prospective randomized trial. Ann Vasc Surg 1992; 6:62-68.

51. Miller A, Marcaccio E, Tannenbaum G et al. Comparison of angioscopy and angiography for monitoring infrainguinal bypass grafts: Results of a

prospective randomized trial. J Vasc Surg 1993; 17: 382.

52. Miller A, Jepsen S, Stonebridge P et al. New angioscopic findings in graft failure after infra-inguinal bypass grafting. Arch Surg 1990; 125:749-55.

53. Fleisher HI, Thompson B, McCowan T et al. Angioscopically monitored saphenous vein valvulotomy. J Vasc Surg 1986; 4:360-364.

54. Matsumoto T, Yang Y, Hashizume M. Direct vision valvulotomy for nonreversed vein graft. Surg Gynecol Obstet 1987; 165:181-183.

55. Mehigan J ed. Angioscopic preparation of the in situ saphenous vein for arterial bypass: Technical considerations. In Angioscopy: vascular and coronary applications, ed. White G, White R, Year Book Medical Publishers Inc, 1989:72-5.

56. Stonebridge P, Miller A, Tsoukas A et al. Angioscopy of arm vein infrainguinal bypass grafts. Ann Vasc Surg 1991; 5:170-175.

57. Marcaccio E, Miller A, Tannenbaum G et al. Angioscopically directed intervention improves arm vein grafts. J Vasc Surg, In press.

58. Salles-Cuhna S, Andros G, Harris R. Preoperative noninvasive assessment of arm veins to be used as bypass grafts in the lower extremities. J Vasc Surg 1986; 3:813-816.

59. Taylor L, Edwards J, Porter J. Present status of reversed vein bypass: Five year results of a modern series. J Vasc Surg 1990; 11:207-215.

CHAPTER 3

PERIOPERATIVE MONITORING

Raul A. Landa

Sushil K. Gupta

Monitoring patency after an arterial reconstruction should start when the patient reaches the recovery room. Assuming that the graft was assessed in the operating room and that this evaluation revealed no abnormality, the entire vascular team should be alert to any sign of graft failure in the early postoperative period because immediate correction of the problem often ensures long-term patency. The reported incidence of graft failure in the postoperative period (30 days) has been between 3% to 18%.[1]

Early failures are usually related to technical factors including: errors in construction of anastomosis, inadequate vein, inadequate outflow, or an unrecognized hypercoagulable state. A good indication of graft patency is the reappearance of pulses in limbs that were not palpable preoperatively. Conversely, the disappearance of pulses that were palpable in the operating room after the revascularization was completed is suggestive of occlusion. Unfortunately, many limbs have residual distal disease and the evaluation of graft patency by clinical means is unreliable and subjective. Also, the presence of a palpable pulse in a graft does not necessarily mean patency because a thrombosed graft can pulsate due to persistent, fluid blood in the graft or incomplete thrombosis. Furthermore, if the graft has been placed in an anatomic position and is deep within the leg, it is almost impossible to palpate the graft.

Both indirect and direct noninvasive testing methods are necessary not only to establish the patency of the bypass graft but also to measure hemodynamic improvement achieved following the infrainguinal bypass. A number of hemodynamic testing methods that can be used to assess the patency of infraingunal reconstructions are described below.

ANKLE BRACHIAL SYSTOLIC PRESSURE INDEX

Measurement of ankle systolic pressure is usually accomplished with a transcutaneous continuous-wave (CW) Doppler. This instrument detects blood flow velocity from the Doppler effect by means of continuous wave transmission of ultrasound into tissue. Back scattered ultrasound is detected and amplified by the instrument as an audible signal. A sphygmomanometer cuff is applied just above the ankle and the Doppler probe is placed over the posterior tibial artery or the dorsalis pedis artery. Flow signals cease as the cuff is inflated above brachial systolic pressure, and during deflation of the cuff a return of flow signal indicates the level of systolic pressure where the cuff is placed. The ankle-brachial systolic pressure index (ABI) is calculated by dividing the pressures between the ankle and the arm. ABI equal to or greater than 0.95 is normal.

This technique used in conjunction with a physical examination of pulses after surgery offers quantitative and objective evaluation of arterial hemodynamics. This exam can be completed in almost all cases except those in which the terminal anastomosis is at foot level or those in which the area around the incision is sensitive thereby making the examination too painful. A normal ABI after surgery or an increase of more than 0.15 compared with the preoperative value is indicative of graft patency and a technically adequate bypass.[2] (Fig. 1)

An abnormal ABI after operation or failure to demonstrate an increase in the index suggest, but does not conclusively establish, the existence of a problem. An abnormal ABI does not predict graft thrombosis or technical error but the level correlates with severity of residual or recurrent limb ischemia. If other evidence is compatible with continued graft function, the ABI should be carefully monitored for the next few hours. Further evaluation such as an arteriogram or reexploration may be delayed until the ABI demonstrates a consistent pattern or if the patient demonstrates renewed signs of ischemia. By contrast, a reduction in the ABI of 0.15 or greater compared with immediate postoperative levels is indicative of occlusion or failing graft.[2,3,4]

Figure 1. Ankle Brachial Systolic Pressure Index before and after left femoral popliteal bypass and angioplasty of a left iliac artery stenosis.

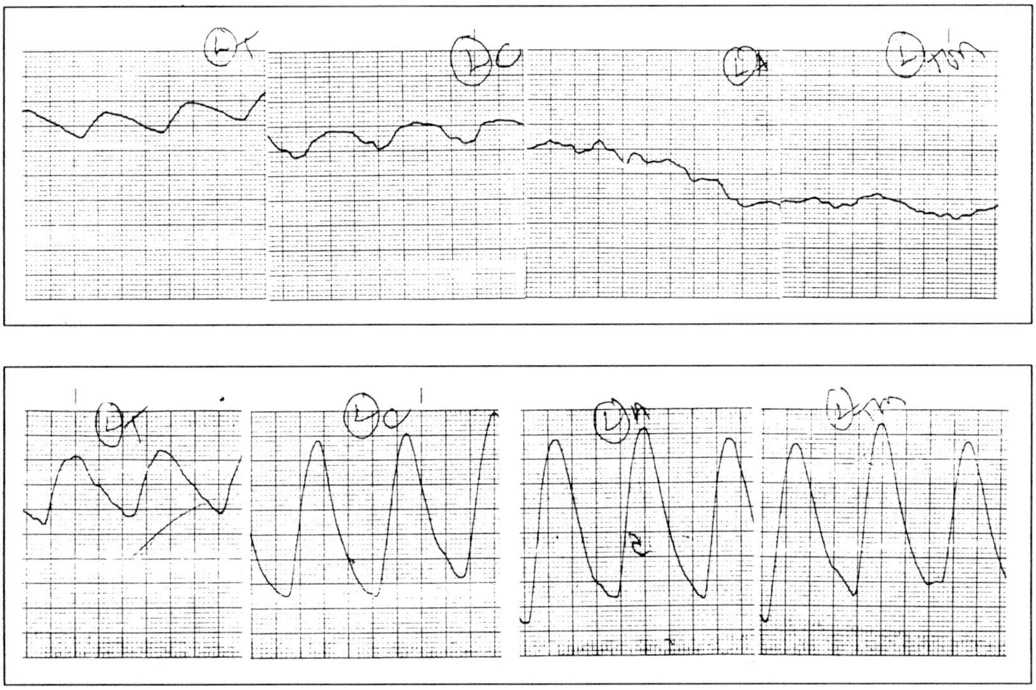

When in-situ saphenous vein grafts have been used and terminate distally in the leg or in some cases of femoropopliteal bypasses, the ABI although improved, may remain low due to the hyperemic phase following revascularization of a severely ischemic extremity. As the hyperemia decreases, the ABI gradually rises.[5]

The disadvantage of this technique is that the pressure measurements alone cannot localize the abnormality or assess whether graft flow has been altered. Also, ABI measurements may be unreliable in 5% to 10% of revascularized limbs due to medial calcification of the peripheral arteries. In addition, the presence of pedal arterial disease may still restrict perfusion of the foot despite adequate inflow pressures. In these cases, other methods of evaluating functional results can be used.

Doppler Flowmeter and Velocity Waveform Analysis or Spectral Analysis of Doppler-Derived Velocity Waveform

Recording of the blood velocity waveform by this technique and evaluation of this waveform is not complicated and is very useful in the immediate postoperative period. Different wave forms can be obtained according to patency or stenosis at different levels of the graft. (Fig. 2) A pulsatile and hyperemic flow often establish graft patency, but absence of a velocity signal or thumping waveform indicates occlusion even when the graft can still pulsate.[5,6]

Unfortunately, only subcutaneous grafts can be accurately assessed with this technique, and the method is most effective in the evaluation of autogenous vein (either in situ or reverse) grafts. A polytetrafluoroethylene graft produces a severe dumping of ultrasound immediately after it has been placed due to air trapped in the interstices of the graft, although later this air is replaced by body fluid and the ultrasound signal can be detected. Umbilical

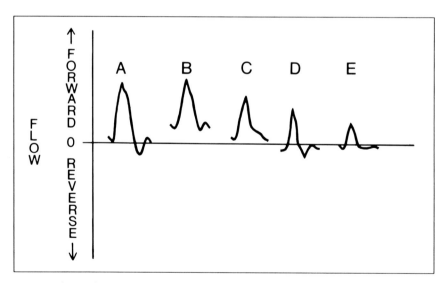

Figure 2. Flow pulse in a vein graft. A. Unobstructed graft with peripheral vasoconstriction. B. Unobstructed graft with peripheral vasodilation. C. Stenosis proximal to the site of the probe. D. Complete obstruction several centimeters distal to the site of the probe. E. Stenosis just below the site of the probe.

veins and Dacron grafts can be evaluated in the immediate postoperative period. Grafts that lie in an anatomic position or that lie deep to the muscle fascia can not be accurately assessed. Duplex scanning is a better alternative for these grafts.

The technique is easily described. A CW Doppler flow detector (5 mHz pulse frequency) is held at a 45 degree angle to the skin. Blood flow patterns are recorded in the mid and the distal graft segments. The back scattered Doppler signal is processed by a real time spectrum analyzer and the velocity spectra is displayed on a video monitor. Blood flow velocity at peak systole (VP) and end diastole (VD) is calculated from operator controlled cursor measurements of the spectra waveform. The magnitude and configuration of the waveform depend on three factors: recording site, time interval after operation, and the outflow resistance of the run-off vessels. A hyperemic flow pattern should be expected in the immediate postoperative period due to an increase in skin temperature and vasodilatation. This pattern usually changes to a triphasic configuration within two months of revascularization.

It is important to remember that the diastolic flow velocity (Vd) decreases during the immediate postoperative period but the peak systolic velocity (Vp) remains constant. The velocity waveform of the distal graft more accurately reflects the hemodynamics of blood flow, especially the level of peripheral vascular resistance. By contrast, the velocity waveform of the proximal graft does not reflect the hemodynamics due to differences in the graft diameter and compliance as both alter the waveform. A peak velocity below 45 cm per second or a drop in peak velocity of 30 cm per second compared to the measurement in the immediate postoperative period indicates a failing graft.[7,8] For this reason, many vascular surgeons have recommended the use of long-term evaluation of patients with infrainguinal bypasses who have a peak systolic velocity (Vp) less than 70 cm per second (around 50% of patients with PTFE bypasses).

The velocity waveform analysis is particularly helpful when evaluating distal bypasses where small veins have to be used. As we know, the small venous conduit can restrict blood flow during the period of revascularization and hyperemia and develop a pressure gradient along the length of the graft. It is important to differentiate this situation from a technical error since high flow velocity is usually present in a small diameter graft segment. If we use this analysis with measurement of immediate postoperative ABI, and remember the normal hemodynamics of the revascularized limb where hyperemia exists, we can avoid further investigation, e.g., angiography and reoperation. Low flow resistance is usually evident by a ratio of end diastolic to peak systolic velocity (Vd/Vp) of greater than 0.25. An abnormal graft velocity waveform after operation should require further investigation with a duplex scan or angiography in order to identify a correctable lesion or an outflow vessel that can accept a sequential bypass to augment graft flow.

DUPLEX SCANNING

Duplex scanning represents the combination of real time B-mode ultrasound imaging and Doppler ultrasound. This technique allows both visualization of a graft and the noninvasive measurement of hemodynamic parameters, i.e., flow and velocity and is discussed in greater detail in Chapters 4 and 5. This noninvasive test has many advantages over other techniques for monitoring patency of infrainguinal bypass, because it has the unique ability to assess both the vascular anatomy as well as physiology. Color has been added to the technique (real time, B mode) that allows rapid survey of anatomic areas for abnormal flow patterns. The addition of color also allows a more precise assignment of Doppler beam angle with respect to the flow field which permits an accurate calculation of flow velocity changes associated with stenosis.[7,9] (Fig. 3)

The advantage of duplex scanning is that it is applicable for surveillance of all infrainguinal bypasses regardless of location (anatomic or subcutaneous) or graft type (vein or prosthetic) Another advantage is that this technique can localize occlusive lesions and categorize their hemodynamic significance over a wide spectrum of stenosis (from minor stenosis to those that need correction). Unfortunately, in the immediate postoperative period, wound tenderness, hematoma, and edema around the graft preclude duplex mapping of the graft. In the case of in situ vein grafts, duplex scanning may be done as early as one day following surgery if there is suspicion of malfunction in the immediate postoperative period . In this setting, use of duplex scanning below the knee is limited to two or three areas of the graft and may detect any significant changes in the velocity waveform. If any difference is found, an angiogram is indicated. No change in velocity may indicate no important abnormalities, but the patient should have a complete duplex scan of the graft before discharge.

The patient is examined in the supine position with the lower extremity externally rotated and the knee bent slightly. In this position, any artery of the leg can be evaluated. The examiner should know what kind of procedure was done, the material used, and the location of the graft as well as the site of anastomosis. The examination is started in the proximal graft and the upper anastomosis is evaluated. In the proximal graft, flow is initially assessed and a triphasic velocity waveform confirms normal inflow; also the presence of a waveform with a pulsatile index greater than 4.0 in the femoral artery is an indication of a abnormal inflow. In the anastomotic sites and graft conduit, one should look for structural abnormalities and site of flow disturbance. Special attention is given to examining the distal anastomosis in several places. The entire lower extremity arterial system and bypass graft require complete duplex mapping when the graft develops a low flow state (peak systolic Vd < 45 cm/sec) or decrease in blood flow velocity (< 30 cm/sec) interval change in Vp.[2,10] Angiography following this finding is usually required.

The advantage of color duplex scanning is that sites of abnormal flow can be recognized early. Changes in maximum blood flow velocity and degree of spectral broadening are indications of abnormal flow and can be classified according to the severity of stenosis.

Usually, a lesion with velocity spectra of greater than 50% stenosis has been associated with an angiographic lesion that needs correction. The only exception to this finding has been a residual valve cusp in a situ saphenous vein bypass graft where the angiogram underestimates the hemodynamic changes.[2]

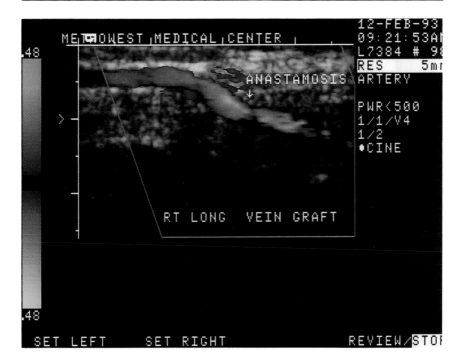

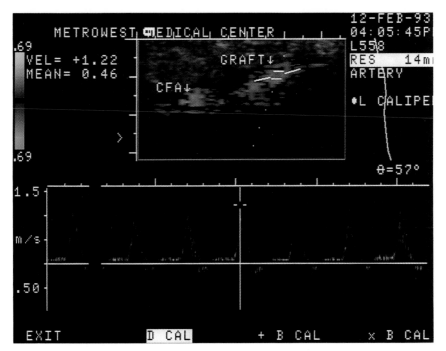

Figure 3. Examples of duplex scanning of graft.

OTHER METHODS OF POSTOPERATIVE MONITORING

CONTINUOUS PIEZOELECTRIC PULSE SENSOR

The pulse amplitude monitor (Paramed Technology, Mountain View, CA) consists of a piezoelectric pulse sensor and display monitor with waveform screen and hard copy printer.[11,12] The piezoelectric pulse sensor generates a signal voltage which is proportional to the pulsatile displacement of the tissue surface overlying the dorsalis pedis artery. The active portion of the sensor is constructed by stretching a 28 cm thick piezoelectric polyvinylidine fluoride foil between raised protrusions on a plastic frame with a tension of 0.9 kg force. Each foil sensor is 27.9 mm long and 13.5 mm wide with an active area of 377 mm. The frame is mounted on a compressible foam block. The dimensions of the shell and material properties of the foam are chosen to press the foil against the tissue with the desired force. When the foil is held firmly against the skin, underlying tissue displacement causes the foil to stretch and relax, generating a charge proportional to the change in foil length. This change is captured in silk-screened silver electrode patterns on both plain surfaces of the foil. The resultant current produces a voltage signal across a resistor which is graphically displayed as a real-time pulsatile waveform on a liquid crystal monitor and can be printed on paper for hard copy. (Fig. 4)

The pulse sensor is taped to the skin over a dorsalis pedis pulse that can be palpated or identified by a Doppler. The process provides the surgeon a continuous, quantitative status of the strength of the pulse. (Fig. 5)

The pulse sensor can be placed immediately before or after surgery, depending on the surgical need for a sterile operating field. The output signal

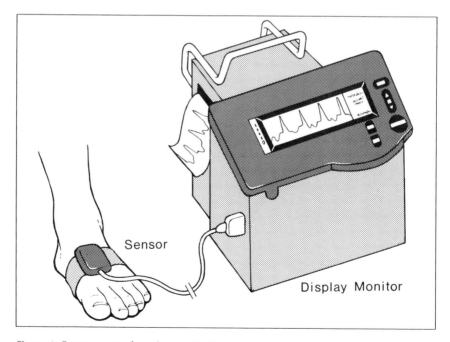

Figure 4. Components of a pulse amplitude monitor

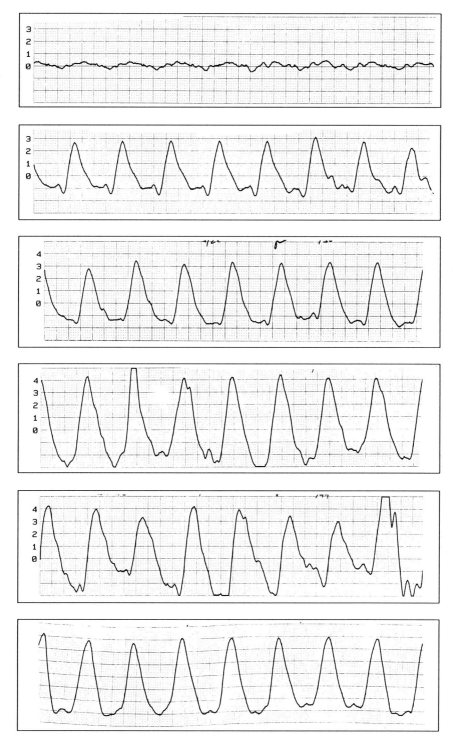

Figure 5. Pre- and postoperative traces of the pulse amplitude monitor in a patient who underwent a femoropopiliteal bypass.

amplification is set at an appropriate gain level and maintained at this setting throughout the study for comparison purposes. The amplitudes are recorded in millimeters, total displacement from the baseline. This continuous monitoring can be inspected by nursing staff at any time and hard copies are produced as needed. This monitoring is usually performed for the first 24 hours after surgery.

After successful infrainguinal revascularization, a uniform, slow rise in amplitude of the piezoelectric waveform over time is expected. The rise in amplitude is independent of both the systolic blood pressure and the pulse pressure and may be related to changes in flow due to a rise or fall in peripheral outflow resistance following reconstruction.

Figure 5 shows the trace of a patient who underwent a femoral-popliteal bypass because of rest pain and a nonhealing ulcer of his left big toe. Figure 5a shows a trace taken preoperatively over the dorsalis pedis artery; the pulse amplitude monitor trace can be seen as almost a flat line. Figure 5b shows the trace minutes after the revascularization was completed. The gain in amplitude was more than 250%. The pulse amplitude monitor was kept on the patient for 24 hours. Figure 5c shows a trace taken at approximately two hours after the graft was completed. Figure 5d shows hard copy taken 24 hours post surgery. The amplitude of the trace is even higher and this is related to a rise in peripheral resistance.

We used this monitoring method successfully in 30 limbs of 33 patients undergoing vascular procedures. Thirteen patients had femoro-popliteal and femoro-distal bypasses and one had a femoral thromboembolectomy. The rest had aorto-iliac surgeries. The piezoelectric sensor was used as described previously. The mean percentage change in amplitude was 320% (range 240-470%.) This increase in amplitude correlated well with the change in ABI done postoperatively (a mean increase of 0.4 from preoperative values).

The piezoelectric pulse sensor monitoring may provide an accurate and objective method to continuously assess limb revascularization in the immediate postoperative period.

References

1. Berkowitz HD. Postoperative screening in peripheral arterial disease. In: Noninvasive diagnostic techniques in vascular disease. Bernstein EF, ed, 3rd edition. 1985: 632-638.
2. Bandyk DF. Postoperative surveillance of Infrainguinal bypass. SCNA 1990; 70: 71-85.
3. Bandyk DF, Seabrook GR, Moldenhauer P et al. Hemodynamics of vein graft stenosis. J Vasc Surg 8: 688-695, 1988.
4. McShane MD, Goddard VM, Clifford PC et al. Duplex ultrasound monitoring of arterial grafts: Prospective evaluation in conjunciton with ankle pressure indices after femorodistal bypass. Eur J Vasc Surg 1987; 1:385-390.
5. Summer DS. Noninvasive assessment of peripheral arterial occlusive disease. In: Vascular Surgery. Rutherford, ed, 3rd edition. 1989: 101-104.
6. Brennan JA, Thrush AJ, Evans DH, Bell PR. Perioperative monitoring of blood flow in femoroinfrangenicullar vein grafts with Doppler ultrasonography: A preliminary report. J Vasc Surg 1991; 13: 468-474.

7. Killevich LA, Fisher CH, Bartlett ST. Surveillance of in situ infrainguinal bypass grafts: conventional vs color flow duplex ultrasonography. J Cardiovasc Surg 1990; 31: 662-667.

8. Bandyk DF, Kalbuick HW, Bergarrini TM et al. Hemodynamics of in situ saphenous vein arterial bypass. Arch Surg 1988; 123: 477.

9. Landrey GL, Hodgson KJ, Spodone DEP et al. Initial experience with color flow dupex scanning of infrainguinal bypass grafts. J Vasc Surg 1990; 12:284-290.

10. Grigg MJ, Wolfe JH, Tovar A, Nicolaides AN. The reliability of duplex derived hemodynamic measurement sin the assessment of femoro-distal grafts. Eur J Vasc Surg 1988; 2: 177-181.

11. Cavaye DM, Tabbara, MR, Kopchok GE, White RA. Continuous Piezoelectric pulse sensor monitoring of peripheral vascular reconstructions. Presented at the Southern California Vascular Surgical Society Annual Scientific Meeting. September, 1991.

12. Gupta SK, Dietzek AM, Veith FJ et al. Use of a piezoelectric film sensor for monitoring vascular grafts. Am J Surg 1990; 160: 182-186.

CHAPTER 4

COMPARISON OF INFRAINGUINAL GRAFT SURVEILLANCE TECHNIQUES

Richard M. Green

Postoperative, noninvasive surveillance can identify hemodynamic abnormalities in infrainguinal bypass grafts.[1] However, the purpose of graft surveillance is not just to identify a stenotic lesion but to predict which graft is at risk for sudden thrombosis. Although the practice of periodic surveillance in the patient with no symptoms has become well established, little data are available on the natural history of such a patient with an untreated hemodynamic abnormality detected on a routine surveillance visit. Proponents of routine graft surveillance argue that identifying an anatomic problem that might lead to graft thrombosis and correcting it should result in improved long-term patency and limb salvage rates.[2,3,4,5] These opinions are based on better secondary patency rates after revision of patent but hemodynamically compromised grafts compared to graft replacement for thrombosis. Since the fate of the hemodynamically compromised but patent grafts in patients with no symptoms is unknown, statistical conclusions comparing primary and secondary patency rates after revision for hemodynamic abnormalities may not be meaningful. Instead, these differences may be due to an arbitrary shift from the primary patency group to the secondary group.

Recently an analysis of the natural history of hemodynamic change in the patient with no symptoms questioned the role of periodic graft surveillance.[6] This study found that significant decreases in the ankle/brachial pressure index (ABI) did not predict graft thrombosis. Others have found that many patients will have graft occlusion without any warning clinical or laboratory signs despite testing.[7] It is therefore important that the natural history of symptomatic hemodynamic changes in infrainguinal grafts be defined. Surveillance protocols must be developed that identify and treat grafts at risk for thrombosis without causing unnecessary interventions. This analysis attempts to do just that by examining the kind of testing that should be performed, the significance of an abnormal result, the frequency of testing, and whether there are factors that should modify this approach.

Reprinted by permission from the Journal of Vascular Surgery.

MATERIAL AND METHODS

We reviewed the records of 300 patients who underwent successful infrainguinal bypass procedures at the University of Rochester Medical Center between January 1983 and December 1987. We established a follow-up graft surveillance protocol that consisted of a patient visit at one month for an ankle pressure measurement and/or a duplex scan and then a visit every six months for the first two years and yearly thereafter. The type of testing was not randomized but was determined by the availability of equipment and personnel. Thirty-eight patients with graft occlusion at one month or earlier were excluded from this review as were 46 patients who did not comply with our follow up protocol. This was usually due to geographic considerations. Thirty-nine patients with recurrent symptoms were evaluated and treated without regard for protocol. One hundred seventy-seven patients with no symptoms met the criteria for the analysis. Ninety-six bypass grafts were placed with in situ saphenous vein, 50 bypass grafts were placed with reversed saphenous vein, and 31 prosthetic bypass grafts were placed (23 expanded polytetrafluoroethylene [ePTFE] and eight umbilical veins.)

Graft surveillances were carried out by certified vascular lab technicians (American Registry of Diagnostic Medical Sonographers, ARDMS) under the supervision of the author. Ankle systolic pressures were determined by the transcutaneous Doppler ultrasonographic flow detection technique by use of an 8 mHz probe. An ABI was calculated based on the higher of the two arm pressures. A stressed ABI was also obtained either by exercising the patient when possible on the treadmill or by creating reactive hyperemia. An ABI was considered abnormal when either the resting or the stressed value was reduced by more than 10% from the previous determination. When this occurred the next follow-up interval was reduced to three months unless recurrent symptoms developed in the patient. Intervals were kept at three months until symptoms occurred or the abnormality was resolved. The 10% value was chosen despite the known biologic and measurement variability in the ABI of 15% to ensure that as many patients as possible with grafts at risk would have positive test results.[8]

Duplex scans were performed on ATL-PV 450 and Mark IV scanners (Advanced Technology Laboratory, Seattle, WA) Morphologic features of the graft and flow abnormalities were evaluated. Peak systolic flow velocity (PSFV) at intervals along the graft and at each anastomosis were calculated. A 5 mHz probe was used for Doppler analysis and a 7.5 mHz probe was used for imaging. An angle of incidence of 60 degrees was used for imaging when possible, or the velocity was corrected to the angle used if 60 degrees could not be obtained. This test was supplemented by a resting ABI determination. The duplex scan outcome was considered abnormal when a structural defect was identified, when the PSFV was less than 40 cm/sec or greater than 120 cm/sec, or when there was a greater than 50% change in the PSFV from the prior examination. If the duplex scan met any of these criteria in a patient with no symptoms, the follow-up interval was shortened to three months. If the patient complained of recurrent symptoms at any time during follow-up, an angiogram was obtained, and the patient was treated appropriately.

Graft thrombosis was the end point of this review and was determined by physical examination, analysis of hemodynamic parameters, angiography, and graft exploration. No graft was revised unless thrombosis or recurrent symptoms occurred. Primary and secondary patency rates were calculated by means of life table analysis.[9] Primary graft patency was defined as a graft that remained patent by clinical and hemodynamic parameters throughout the period of observation without intervention. Secondary patency was defined as a patent graft after a successful operative intervention for thrombosis or recurrent symptoms.

Conditional probabilities were determined for each test based on the above criteria for normal and abnormal. A test was considered successful if it was normal and the patient did not suffer a graft thrombosis before the next visit. A test failed if it was normal but a graft thrombosis developed in the patient. The sensitivity, or the probability that a graft abnormality tests positive, and specificity, the probability that a normal graft tests negative, were calculated. The predictive values of a positive and negative test were also determined.[10]

RESULTS

LIFE TABLE ANALYSIS OF GRAFT PATENCY

Eighteen graft thromboses (10%) occurred in this series over the 5-year period of observation. Successful revision was accomplished in 9 of the 18 thrombosed grafts (50%). Recurrent symptoms prompted graft revision in 20 patients (11%), and 18 of these secondary operations were successful (90%). Twenty-nine of the 38 revisions were necessary within the first 18 months, and 17 of the revisions were necessary in the 6- to 12-month interval. The primary and secondary cumulative patency rates (CPRs) are shown in Figure 1

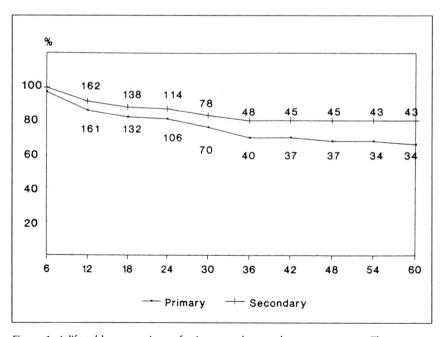

Figure 1. A life table comparison of primary and secondary patency rates. These curves represent grafts that were revised only for thrombosis or recurrent symptoms.

and Tables 1 and 2. The one-year primary CPR was 86% compared to a secondary CPR of 91%. The five-year primary CPR was 66% compared to a secondary CPR of 80%.

Table 1. Life table analysis of primary graft patency

Months of observation	Ox	Dx	Wx	Qx	px	Px
0-6	177	5	11	0.03	0.97	0.97
>6-12	161	17	12	0.11	0.89	0.86
>12-18	132	7	19	0.05	0.95	0.82
>18-24	106	1	35	0.01	0.99	0.81
>24-30	70	4	26	0.06	0.94	0.76
>30-36	40	2	1	0.05	0.95	0.70
>36-42	37	0	0	0.00	1.00	0.70
>42-48	37	1	2	0.03	0.97	0.68
>48-54	34	0	0	0.00	1.00	0.68
>54-60	34	1	5	0.03	0.97	0.66

Ox Patient under observation beginning of interval
Dx Thrombosed or withdrawn for revision as a result of symptoms during interval
Wx Withdrawn patient during interval
Qx Chance of interval failure
px Chance of interval success
Px Cumulative chance of success

Table 2. Life table analysis of secondary graft patency

Months of observation	Ox	Dx	Wx	Qx	px	Px
0-6	177	1	11	0.005	0.995	0.995
>6-12	162	12	12	0.075	0.925	0.915
>12-18	138	5	19	0.04	0.96	0.88
>18-24	114	1	35	0.01	0.99	0.87
>24-30	78	4	26	0.05	0.95	0.83
>30-36	48	2	1	0.04	0.96	0.80
>36-42	45	0	0	0.00	1.00	0.80
>42-48	45	0	2	0.00	1.00	0.80
>48-54	43	0	0	0.00	1.00	0.80
>54-60	43	0	5	0.00	1.00	0.80

Ox Patient under observation beginning of interval
Dx Thrombosed during interval
Wx Withdrawn patient during interval
Qx Chance of interval failure
px Chance of interval success
Px Cumulative chance of success

THE ANKLE/BRACHIAL INDEX

The ABI with either exercise or reactive hyperemia was performed alone on 428 occasions. A value within 10% of the prior determination was obtained in 338 tests in 82 different patients. Sudden graft thrombosis occurred before the next scheduled visit in five of these patients (1.4%). Four of these patients had ePTFE grafts, and this accounted for four of the six graft occlusions in the 23 patients with ePTFE. One patient had an in situ saphenous vein graft, which failed between the 6 to 12 month interval without any warning signs or symptoms. A decrease of 10% or more from the prior determination occurred on 90 examinations in 68 different patients with no symptoms. (Fig. 2) Graft surveillance intervals were then decreased to three months, and the abnormality persisted in 26 patients. Angiograms were obtained for 20 of these patients with symptoms. Correctable lesions were identified in eight patients whose grafts were revised. Angioplasties of the outflow artery were required in four of these patients, distal sequential bypasses where placed in two patients, and inflow procedures were performed in the other two patients. Four of the other 12 patients had inoperable outflow occlusions with patent grafts, five had graft thrombosis and three had no obvious lesion. Three of the four patients with outflow occlusions had graft thrombosis within six months. None of the patients with normal angiographic results had graft thrombosis. No further studies were performed in the six patients who remained asymptomatic despite a persistent decrease in their ABI. Sudden graft occlusion developed in three of these patients before their next visit, and the other three have remained patent. In total, 19 of these 26 patients with persistently abnormal ABI values required either revision for thrombosis or for symptoms during the study period.

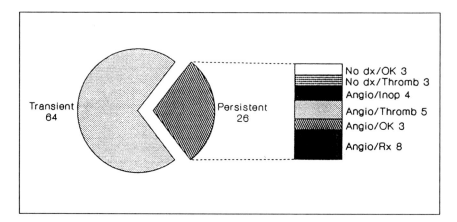

Figure 2. The fate of an abnormal ABI (0.10 decrease). An abnormal ABI in the absence of symptoms promoted a decrease in the surveillance interval to 3 months. The abnormality persisted in 26 patients. No further diagnostic tests (No Dx) were done in six patients and three grafts failed before the next visit (no Dx/Thromb). Angiograms were obtained for 20 patients in whom symptoms developed. Correctable lesions (Angio/Rx) were identified and fixed in eight patients, normal grafts were identified in three patients (Angio/OK), graft thromboses were seen in five patients (Angio/Throm), and inoperable outflow lesions were seen in four patients (Angio/inop).

Table 3. Test results

Result	No. of observations	Thrombosis or symptoms
Normal ABI	338	5 (1.5%)
Normal duplex/normal ABI	273	0 (0%)*
Abnormal ABI	90	10 (11%)
Abnormal duplex/normal ABI	106	4 (4%)**
Abnormal duplex/abnormal ABI	29	19 (66%)***

*The combination of a normal duplex scan outcome and ABI is better for identifying normal grafts than an ABI alone.
**An abnormal ABI is better than an abnormal duplex scan outcome in detecting a graft at risk for thrombosis.
***An abnormal ABI and an abnormal duplex scan outcome is better than an abnormal ABI alone for detecting a graft at risk for thrombosis.

THE DUPLEX SCAN

Scans were performed at 408 surveillance visits in conjunction with ABI measurements. There were 273 occasions where both the scan results and ABI value were normal. No patient with these findings suffered a sudden graft occlusion before the next scheduled visit. One hundred six surveillances in 53 patients resulted in an abnormal duplex scan outcome but a normal ABI value. Four of these patients had a sudden graft thrombosis before their next visit. All four of these patients had PSVF greater than 12 cm/sec at the distal anastomoses of an in situ saphenous vein bypass graft to a tibial artery. On 29 occasions both the duplex scan outcome and the ABI values were abnormal. Sudden graft thrombosis occurred in 19 of these patients before the next scheduled visit. Follow-up intervals were decreased to three months in the other 10 patients, and the abnormalities persisted without graft thrombosis. But recurrent symptoms occurred in six patients who required an inflow operation.

The ABI is a very important accompanying test to the duplex scan. When the ABI is normal and the duplex scan outcome is abnormal as described herein, the risk of graft occlusion is only 4% over the next three months. When the ABI is reduced 10% or more and the duplex scan finding is abnormal, the risk of graft occlusion is 66%. Table 3 shows the incidence of interval graft thrombosis after each test and the conditional probabilities of thrombosis by use of the criteria above for normal and abnormal.

STATISTICAL EVALUATION

The specificity, sensitivity and predictive value of a positive test and predictive value of a negative test were calculated. (Fig. 3) The sensitivity or the probability that a graft was about to occlude within the next follow-up interval will yield a positive test outcome was only 66% for the ABI alone but was 100% for the duplex scan with and without an abnormal ABI. the specificity or the probability that a nonthreatened graft will yield a negative test was 80% for the ABI alone, 72% for the duplex alone and 96% for the duplex combined with an ABI. The predictive value for an abnormal ABI is 12%, 4% for an abnormal duplex scan outcome, and 65% when both the duplex scan result and the ABI value are abnormal. The predictive value of a normal ABI was 98% and 100% for the duplex scan with and without an abnormal ABI.

DISCUSSION

No one would deny the importance of revising an infrainguinal bypass graft when a patient returns with ischemic symptoms and reduced arterial hemodynamics. Abundant data exist that show long-term patency rates are improved when patent grafts with hemodynamically significant stenoses are revised before thrombosis compared to grafts that are revised or replaced after thrombosis.[11,12] It is only natural that vascular surgeons would therefore diligently look for grafts with stenoses in patients with no symptoms to avoid thrombosis and the poorer results that follow replacement in that situation. An assumption was made that long-term patency rates would improve if all preocclusive lesions were identified and treated even though the patient did not complain of symptoms.[13] Data are nonexistent about the natural history of these "preocclusive lesions" that have been revised in patients with no symptoms. Is it fair to arbitrarily reduce the primary patency rates by elimi- nating all patients with reduced ABIs or abnormal duplex scan results, revising these grafts and saying that the secondary curves are really better? Will a high proportion of these grafts actually thrombose if revision is not

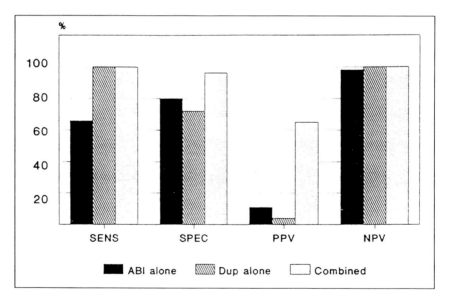

Figure 3. Conditional probabilities for the tests with stated norms. The sensitivity (SENS) or the probability that a graft about to occlude will yield a positive test was highest for the duplex scan with or without the ABI. The specificity (SPEC) or the probability that a nonthreatened graft will test normally was highest when both the duplex and the ABI were normal. The predictive value of an abnormal test (PPV) was highest for the combination of an abnormal duplex and ABI. The predictive value of a negative test (NPV) was similar for all the tests.

carried out? This study was conducted to determine the fate of the graft in the patient with no symptoms when a policy was adopted to only revise grafts when symptoms occur.

Deterioration of the postoperative ABI is correlated with angiographic documentation of flow restricting lesions in the graft or host arteries.[14] We used a change of greater than 0.10 as significant even though others use a change of 0.15 to 0.20 because of the known biologic variability of this ratio. We acknowledge that by using this relatively low value we may have biased the results adversely. However, even with this allowance five grafts with normal ABI values thrombosed before the next surveillance visit. Four of the five were ePTFE grafts, and one was an in situ saphenous vein graft. O'Donnell et al[15] also found ABI a poor indicator of ePTFE grafts about to thrombose.

The ABI was reduced after 90 examinations, but the value returned to normal range on 64 occasions. This variability accounted for the lower sensitivity and predictive value of an abnormal ABI. When the ABI remained abnormal three months later it took on a new significance because grafts in 19 of these 26 patients either thrombosed or required a revision because recurrent symptoms developed. It would follow then that a reduced ABI, which persists three months even in the absence of symptoms should portend graft failure and prompt prophylactic action. The limitation in this approach is that 8 of the 11 grafts that thrombosed in this group of 19 patients did so before the next surveillance visit. Barnes et al[16] followed patients with no symptoms with resting ABI reduced by 0.2 or more and found that this reduction in postoperative ABI did not predict impending graft thrombosis. Our data which used a lower value of ABI change would suggest that a persistently abnormal ABI documents but does not predict graft thrombosis.

Duplex scanning has been recently used to assess hemodynamic and structural changes in femoropopliteal bypass grafts. Bandyk et al[17] recognized that 20-40% of grafts that thrombosed did so with a normal ABI, and that an abnormal ABI did not necessarily identify grafts at risk for thrombosis. They determined that Doppler derived peak systolic blood flow velocities of less than 45 cm/sec identified grafts with impending failure. Although our study did not deal with grafts in the early postoperative period we agree with these authors about the need for immediate graft flow analysis with the duplex scanner for identification of the immediate problems such as incomplete valve lysis in an in situ vein graft, which leads to graft thrombosis.

Bandyk et al[18] reported that an aggressive policy of revising grafts with hemodynamic abnormalities resulted in similar four-year CPRS for nonrevised (86%) and revised (81%) in situ grafts. They revised 70 of the 250 grafts (28%) followed. The decrease in ABI in their revised grafts averaged 0.24 but 34% of all patients had values less than 0.20. They concluded from these data that revision of these hemodynamically compromised grafts even in a patient with no symptoms would minimize the chance of graft thrombosis and therefore improve the overall result. However, there is a conceptual problem with comparing these primary and secondary life table curves when one arbitrarily removes patent grafts from the primary life table on the basis of velocity abnormalities. These are really the same patients in two samples from two independent populations. This is really a before and after situation. There must be a difference in the two curves unless the revisions all failed, and that is obviously not the case. The difference in the two curves should not be looked at statistically because the natural history of the patent graft with hemodynamic abnormalities is unknown. If each revised graft would fail without revision then the difference between the two curves would indicate the benefit of revision. On the other hand, if only a small fraction of the patent grafts would thrombose, there would be little benefit of prophylactic revision.

At the onset of this study we questioned whether all grafts with velocity changes require revision when the patient has no symptoms. When a policy of operating only on patients with symptoms was followed, we found that 38 of 177 (21.5%) grafts required revision, and that 18 of those grafts already had thrombosed. The total failure rate of 21.5% in this series is similar to the 28% failure rate reported by Bandyk et al.[18] The cumulative secondary patency rate of 80% in our series is similar to the 85% rate in the study by Bandyk et al[4] at four years. The striking difference between the two series is that 18 (47%) of our "graft failures" were actually thromboses, whereas only 10 (10%) of the failures in the series of Bandyk et al[18] were thrombosed at the time of revision. We now believe based on the results of this study that certain hemodynamic abnormalities in patients with no symptoms do portend graft thrombosis and should be acted on when identified. Our data indicate that when the duplex scan results and the ABI are abnormal that the risk of graft thrombosis is high (66% within three months), and that revision even in a patient with no symptoms is indicated. Failure to do so means that one is faced with a thrombosed graft that requires thrombolytic therapy and revision under compromised circumstances as opposed to a patent graft with a stenosis. We found that an abnormally increased PSFV is just as serious a flow abnormality as an abnormally low peak flow when combined with a reduced ABI. We were fortunate that we were successful in achieving as good a secondary patency rate as we did, as others have not been as successful in these circumstances.

The incidence of graft thrombosis in the interval after an abnormal duplex scan in the setting of a normal ABI is low and is a reason to decrease surveillance intervals but not necessarily an indication to proceed to arteriography. The four patients in our series who had graft thrombosis all had elevated flows at the distal anastomoses of tibial artery in situ grafts. We would not quarrel with decreasing the surveillance interval to even less than three months in patients with high risk grafts and duplex abnormalities.

The time course and causes of graft thrombosis are well documented,[19] and surveillance protocols should be timed to identify grafts in trouble during high risk periods. The risk of graft thrombosis is highest in the first 30 days, and immediate postoperative evaluation is therefore necessary. We now recommend follow up at one month and then every three months for the first year, every six months for the next year, and yearly thereafter unless a hemodynamic abnormality exists. If the ABI or the duplex scan result is abnormal the surveillance interval is decreased to three months, if the ABI and duplex scan outcomes are abnormal an arteriogram is obtained.

This study attempted to define the natural history of the patient with no symptoms with a hemodynamic abnormality in an infrainguinal bypass graft. It was a retrospective and nonrandomized analysis and is therefore not of the most rigorous design to accomplish this task.[20] This was a study of graft surveillance techniques not graft materials. Therefore, the inclusion of synthetic grafts had little impact on the analysis. Nonetheless, this review does show that certain hemodynamic conditions in infrainguinal bypass grafts portend graft thrombosis. If one fails to act on a graft with both a reduced ABI and abnormally high or low flow velocities, one risks graft thrombosis before the next follow up visit. Revision under these circumstances is less likely to be successful than revision of a patent graft. On the other hand, one need not act if these conditions do not exist. Flow abnormalities without pressure drops may be quite stable over time and can be observed with more frequent testing for further changes or the development of symptoms. Pressure drops in the absence of flow abnormalities are apt to be variable, and although they should be monitored frequently they do not necessarily indicate impending graft thrombosis.

REFERENCES

1. Turnipseed WD, Archer CW. Postoperative surveillance: An effective means of detecting correctable lesions that threaten graft patency. Arch Patients 1985; 120:324-8.
2. Bandyk DF, Schmitt DD, Seabrook GR et al. Monitoring functional patency of in situ saphenous vein bypasses: The impact of a surveillance protocol and elective revision. J Vasc Surg 1989; 9:286-96.
3. Smith CR, Green RM, DeWeese JA. Pseudoocclusion of femoropopliteal bypass grafts. Circulation 1983; 68(suppl II):88-93.
4. Bandyk DF, Kaebnick HW, Stewart GW et al. Durability of the in situ saphenous vevein bypass arterial bypass: A comparison of primary and secondary patency. J Vasc Surg 1987;5:256-68.
5. Green RM, Ouriel K, Ricotta JR et al. Revision of failed infrainguinal bypass graft: principles of management. Surgery 1986; 100:646-53.
6. Barnes RW, Thompson BW, Macdonald CM et al. Serial noninvasive studies do not herald postoperative failure of femoropopliteal or femorotibial bypass grafts. Ann Surg. 1989; 210(4): 486-494.
7. Blackshear WM Jr, Thiele BL, Strandness, DE Jr. Natural history of above and below-knee femoropopliteal grafts. Am J Surg 1980;140:234-41.
8. Baker DJ, Dix D. Variability of Doppler ankle pressure with arterial occlusive disease: An evaluation of ankle index and brachial-ankle pressure gradient. Surgery 1981;89:134-7.
9. Dunn, OJ. Basic statistics. 2nd ed. New York: John Wiley & Sons, 1964:178-87.
10. Ingelfinger, JA, Mosteller F. Thibodeau LA et al. Biostatistics in clinical medicine, 2nd ed. New York: MacMillan, 1987:7-10.
11. Cohen RJ, Mannick JA, Couch NP et al. Recognition and management of impending vein-graft failure. Arch Surg 1986;121:758-9.
12. Bartlett ST, Olinde AJ, Flinn WR et al. The reoperative potential of infrainguinal bypass: Long-term limb and patient survival. J Vasc Surg 1987;5:170-9.
13. Bertkowitz HD, Hobbs CL, Roberts B et al. Value of routine vascular laboratory studies to identify vein graft stenosis. Surgery 1981;90:971-9.
14. O'Mara CS, Flinn, WR, Johnson ND et al. Recognition and surgical management of failing lower extremity arterial reconstruction prior to graft occlusion. J. Cardiovasc Surg [Torino] 1984;25:381-4.

15. O'Donnell TF Jr, Mackey W, McCullough JL et al. Correlation of operative findings with angiographic and noninvasive hemodynamic factors associated with failure of polytetrafluoroethylene grafts. Ann Surg (Unpublished data).

16. Barnes RW, Thompson BW, MacDonald CM et al. Serial noninvasive studies do not herald postoperative failure of femoropopliteal or femorotibial bypass grafts. Surgery 1985;98:799-809.

17. Bandyk DF, Cato RF, Towne JB. A low velocity profile predicts failure of femoropopliteal and femorotibial bypass grafts. Surgery 1985;98:799-809.

18. Bandyk DF, Schmitt DD, Seabrook GR et al. Monitoring functional patency of in situ saphenous vein bypasses: the impact of a surveillance protocol and elective revision. J Vasc Surg 1989;9:286-95.

19. DeWeese JA, Green RM. Anastomotic neointimal fibrous hyperplasia. In: Bernhard VM, Towne JB eds. Complications in vascular surgery. New York: Grune & Stratton, 1980: 153-70.

20. Barnes RW. Understanding investigative clinical trials. J Vasc Surg 1989;9:609-18.

DUPLEX MONITORING OF THE VASCULAR GRAFT

Dennis F. Bandyk

Vascular laboratory surveillance of arterial grafts for occlusive or aneurysmal lesions that threaten graft patency is a generally accepted but unproven concept in vascular surgery. Although a number of retrospective[1-4] and prospective[5-10] observational studies have confirmed improved assisted primary patency following institution of a graft surveillance protocol, many vascular surgeons have not recommended graft monitoring to their patients. The majority continue to rely on clinical evaluation alone or coupled with measurements of ankle systole pressure to detect the "hemodynamically-failing" graft. Reluctance to institute a formal graft surveillance protocol appears to be based on several concerns including: the efficacy of graft revision in an asymptomatic patient, reimbursement for vascular testing, and increased vascular laboratory workload. Barnes et al[11] questioned the efficacy of graft surveillance when no benefit was demonstrated in postoperative patients using changes in ankle-brachial systolic pressure index (ABI) as an endpoint. Graft failure rates were similar (approximately 60%) in patients with stable and recently decreased (>0.2) ABIs. Many of these voiced concerns can only be addressed by a randomized, prospective clinical trial on graft surveillance.[12] The logistics of such a clinical trial are significant and beyond the scope of single institution. Thus at present, each individual surgeon must ascertain the merits of graft surveillance and institute a program based on the resources available.

The goal of graft surveillance is not only to detect lesions with a potential for precipitating graft thrombosis but also to provide surgeons with parameters which identify those grafts at highest risk and thus should undergo a secondary revision procedure. Depending on the graft type (autologous vein, prosthetic) and runoff arteries, graft failure rates in excess of 30% at five years are commonplace. There is convincing evidence that autologous vein graft strictures detected by both angiography and duplex scanning are associated with a significantly increased risk of graft occlusion in comparison to normal grafts. Grigg et al[13] and Moody et al[14] observed a 21-23% incidence of graft thrombosis in stenotic bypasses when a conservative no revision policy was followed. In a recent report by Buth et al[15] all vein grafts identified to have a >70% diameter reduction stenosis, occluded. This is compared to 10% in grafts with similar lesions but revised (p<0.004). Mattos et al[16] also recently reported that infrainguinal grafts identified to have a stenosis by color duplex scanning had a significantly lower four-year patency of 57% compared to 83% observed in normal grafts. Revision of a stenotic graft without interruption in patency is particularly important for autologous vein conduits because most will not remain patent following thrombectomy/thrombolysis alone or with vein-patch angioplasty. Five-year graft patencies in the range of 30-50% have been observed following secondary procedures on thrombosed grafts, as compared to assisted primary patencies of 82-93% following stenosis repair in patent bypasses.[17,18] Based on available clinical data, it appears graft surveillance is beneficial and associated with a 10-15% increase in assisted primary patency rates. At present, graft surveillance protocols should be considered in an evolutionary phase, but some recommendations regarding testing methods/intervals and diagnostic criteria are possible based on the known temporal patterns and mechanism of graft failure. The "best" program for surveillance has not beeen validated and most investigators have adopted a policy of "selective" secondary intervention when a graft stenosis is identified by changes in ABI, duplex scanning, or arteriography. The rationale for graft surveillance is based on the hypothesis that careful monitoring of graft/limb hemodynamics can decrease the observed steady decline in patency of arterial grafts by identifying those grafts which harbor lesions and should undergo elective revision. Those advocating graft surveillance must remain cognizant of costs and develop protocols which minimize frequency of testing but yield positive results.

Mechanisms of Graft Failure

Graft failure can occur by three mechanisms: occlusion by thrombosis, hemodynamic failure, and structural failure, i.e., aneurysmal degeneration. Following operation, the frequency of graft failure is highest within the first 10-14 days (4-10%), decreases to approximately 1% per month during the first year, and then is approximately 2-4% per year thereafter. The timing of graft failure usually predicts the underlying mechanism. Perioperative (within 30 days) failure is most commonly due to technical errors in bypass construction (suture stenosis, intimal flaps, retained thrombus, graft entrapment/torsion). The incidence of early graft failure can be minimized by careful intraoperative assessment, but uncommon mechanisms, such as congenital or acquired hypercoagulable states, use of marginal sclerotic venous conduits, low cardiac output, and poor outflow tracts account for sporadic early graft thrombosis despite a technically perfect reconstruction. Infrainguinal bypasses, especially prosthetic grafts, with poor runoff can demonstrate a blood flow velocity near the "thrombotic threshold velocity" of the conduit and thus be prone to thrombosis with slight decreases in blood flow.

Following operation, a number of abnormalities can persist unsuspected following infrainguinal vein bypass grafting, especially when the in situ saphenous vein grafting technique has been utilized. Retained valve cusps, errors in tunnelling, vein conduit injury, or partial anastomotic occlusion can reduce graft flow to very low levels and precipitate thrombosis. Residual lesions can also be foci for the subsequent development of myointimal hyperplasia, a lesion which when progressive is a known cause of graft failure during the first two years after operation. Postimplantation lesions have been identified in 11-33% of saphenous vein grafts using either angiography or duplex scanning, with approximately 75% developing within the first postoperative year.[2,6,8,15,18] The pathogenesis and prevention of myointimal hyperplasia is an active area of vascular research with anatomic, hemodynamic, and cellular growth factors implicated in its pathobiology.

Atherosclerosis also can develop de novo in vein grafts or progress in adjacent native arteries and produce late graft failure. This mechanism of failure tends to occur after the second postoperative year in autologous vein bypasses but has been observed earlier following polytetrafluorethylene (PTFE) bypass grafting thrombosis, typically with involvement of the distal artery tree. Structural failure is an uncommon mode of late graft thrombosis and usually manifests as aneurysmal degeneration. The mechanism of graft thrombosis involves accumulation of mural thrombus within the aneurysmal segment leading to occlusion or distal embolization. This mode of failure should be suspected when thrombosis occurs despite normal graft surveillance studies. Occlusive lesions, such as technical errors, acquired myointimal graft stenosis, or atherosclerotic disease progression produce graft thrombosis by decreasing blood velocity below a minimal velocity at which thrombus formation can ensue.[19] Duplex scanning, by providing objective data on hemodynamics, can identify the subgroup of grafts with low velocity hemodynamics. Grafts with abnormal hemodynamics appear to be at increased risk for thrombosis. Green et al[4] reporting on a retrospective comparison of graft surveillance techniques found grafts harboring lesions that decreased ankle-brachial systolic pressure index (ABI) by 10% or greater and had an abnormal duplex scan (low graft velocity and/or stenosis) had a 66% incidence of thrombosis within three months, compared with 14% risk of failure if only the ABI was abnormal, and 4% risk of failure if only the duplex scan was abnormal.

Based on the mechanisms of graft failure and the propensity of autologous vein grafts to develop intrinsic lesions, serial duplex scanning has been advocated for postoperative surveillance. This approach is associated with expense, is time-consuming, and requires a level of expertise which may not be available in all hospitals/clinics. Arteriography, like duplex scanning, is a diagnostic imaging technique capable of identifying a spectrum of lesions of which only a portion place the graft at risk for sudden thrombosis. The relationship between degree of stenosis detected by duplex scanning/arteriography and risk of thrombosis requires further study. Recent studies indicate high-grade (>70% diameter reduction) stenoses with end-diastolic velocity greater than 100 cm/sec demonstrate a high correlation with graft thrombosis. By contrast, use of a single criteria, such as peak systolic velocity <45 cm/sec in a normal graft segment or a decrease in ABI, is associated with a low positive predictive value for unexpected graft thrombosis. Prospective graft surveillance programs have confirmed that development of a low velocity graft state, particularly if prior testing demonstrated normal graft velocity, is a harbinger of thrombosis and should prompt complete imaging of the lower limb arterial circulation to delineate sites of stenosis.[3,5,7] Color duplex imaging, if available, is the best initial technique for bypass imaging, although incomplete evaluation of inflow and runoff vessels limits its effectiveness in some patients. In selected patients, i.e., those with a high-grade stenosis identified in the main body of the graft or at an anastomosis and low graft flow velocity/ABI, duplex scanning can supplant arteriography for clinical decision making on the need for graft revision. I have found serial evaluation of graft hemodynamics offers several advantages: it gauges initial technical success, identifies deterioration in graft function at a time when developing occlusive lesions may be easily managed by elective surgical revision or percutaneous transluminal angioplasty. Equally important, it documents the hemodynamic benefit of graft revision, i.e., normalization of graft velocity.[20]

A wide range of duplex-derived blood velocities have been measured in infrainguinal grafts following successful bypass grafting (Table 1).[21] In general, peak systolic velocity in the mid-distal graft segments exceeds 40-45 cm/sec unless the conduit diameter is greater than 6 mm or the graft runoff is limited (isolated tibial artery segment, dorsalis pedis artery bypass). Belkin et al[22] demonstrated peak systolic velocity varies with luminal diameter and recommended duplex surveillance scans of vein grafts be performed using diameter-specific criteria. Of note, these authors found graft velocity was lower (p<0.04) in inframalleolar grafts (59 cm/sec) compared to tibial (77 cm/sec) and popliteal (71 cm/sec) grafts. Only 4 of 72 grafts, all to inframalleolar arteries, had a peak systolic velocity below 45 cm/sec measured. Use of arm vein (cephalic, basilic) or varicose saphenous segments is also associated with low graft conduit velocity, but this hemodynamic observation by itself does not indicate impending thrombosis, but may serve as an indication for postoperative anticoagulation. When normal-sized (3-6 mm diameter) venous conduits are utilized, identification of a graft velocity below 40-45 cm/sec is uncommon, during or following operation. In my experience, this has

Table 1. Peak systolic flow velocity of femoropopliteal and femortibial grafts

Graft Type	No.	Flow velocity (cm/sec)
In situ saphenous vein		
Femoropopliteal	60	76 ± 12
Femorotibial	81	70 ± 16
Femoropopliteal Isolated segment	8	66 ± 15
Reversed saphenous vein		
Femoropopliteal	18	80 ± 16
PTFE, 6 mm diameter		
Femoropopliteal	31	71 ± 14
Femorotibial	28	60 ± 12
PTFE, 5 mm diameter		
Femorotibial	4	78 ± 10

Blood flow velocity was calculated 1 to 3 months after surgery.
Flow velocities are mean standard deviations.
PTFE-Polytetrafluoroethylene (Gore-tex)

Table 2. Categories of graft blood flow patterns

Duplex Category	Velocity Spectra (Waveform) Characteristics
Normal	
Normal PVR	Triphasic configuration, Vp> 45 cm/sec at mid distal graft recording site. Applicable for vein diameter 3-5 mm.
Low PVR	Biphasic configuration, end diastolic flow velocity >0, Vp > 45 cm/sec; an expected waveform at operation and in early postoperative period.
Abnormal, low flow velocity	
High PVR	Monophasic configuration, no diastolic forward flow, Vp < 45 cm/sec. ABI typically between 0.7 and 0.9.
	Stacato Doppler signal with flow reversal during diastole, Vp < 45 cm/sec, minimum antegrade flow due to high grade distal stenosis.
Low PVR	Biphasic waveform with Vp< 45 cm/sec or greater than 30 cm/sec decrease compared to prior level. Compensatory diastolic fllow due to abnormal ABI (0.4-0.7).

PVR-peripheral vascular resistance
Vp-peak systolic velocity

correlated with a residual graft lesion in the perioperative period, or an acquired lesion if measured during follow-up. Low graft velocity due to poor runoff is an infrequent finding and when it occurs is usually based on angiographic assessment of the runoff vessels and the presence of low systolic and diastolic flow despite severe foot ischemia. When a low flow state is identified, a prompt and thorough graft evaluation should ensue, especially if ABI is abnormal (<0.9). Management of low velocity grafts due to poor runoff is controversial but options include: anticoagulation, sequential bypass grafting, or adjunctive distal arteriovenous fistula; the latter two modalities are constructed to augment graft flow.

The velocity spectra used to monitor vascular grafts can be classified into two normal and three abnormal categories. (Table 2) In limbs revascularized for critical ischemia, a hyperemic flow pattern is normally recorded from the graft in the perioperative period. (Fig. 1) Antegrade flow throughout the pulse cycle reflects low peripheral vascular resistance and correlates with signs of revascularization hyperemia (skin warmth, vasodilatation). Within days to several weeks, hyperemia dissipates and the velocity waveform evolves to a triphasic configuration, typically of normal peripheral artery flow and associated with normalization of the ABI.

Transformation of the normal triphasic graft velocity waveform to a biphasic or monophasic configuration coupled with a decrease in peak systolic velocity is highly diagnostic of a remote occlusive lesion. Three waveform configurations have been observed with the development of a graft stenosis which is pressure- and flow-reducing. (Fig. 2) All were associated

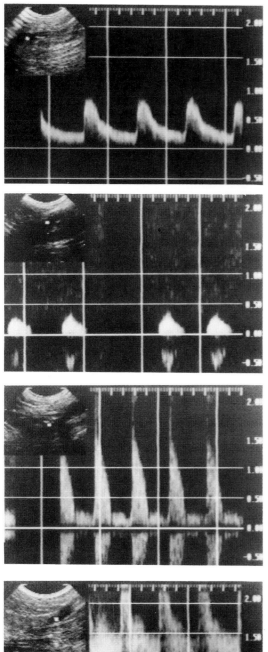

Figure 1. Normal graft flow patterns. Serial velocity spectra recorded from the distal segment of a femorotibial in situ saphenous vein (3.5 mm diameter) graft. Note peak systolic velocity remained constant during this time interval.

Figure 2a-c. Velocity spectra and hemodynamic characteristics of three abnormal graft flow patterns observed with the development of graft stenosis.

with a low (<45 cm/sec) or decrease (> 30 cm/sc compared to prior testing) in peak systolic flow velocity. The most common abnormal graft waveform, present in approximately one-half of cases, was biphasic in configuration and associated with a resting ABI of 0.4-0.7. The forward diastolic flow was in response to compensatory arteriolar dilatation. The site of graft stenosis may be proximal or distal to the recording site. A monophasic waveform with low peak systolic velocity has been observed in approximately 40% of grafts with stenosis. All patients were asymptomatic and resting ABI varied from 0.7 to 0.9. Typically the severity of stenosis was classified in the 50-75% diameter reduction category by both duplex scanning and arteriography. A uncommon (6% of abnormal grafts) but ominous waveform demonstrated a staccato velocity spectra representing to-and-fro motion of blood within the compliant venous conduit with each pulse cycle. This waveform is always associated with a high-grade distal graft stenosis and is a harbinger of graft thrombosis. The minimal antegrade flow in these grafts complicate angiographic visualization of the distal graft and anastomosis, sometimes termed "pseudoocclusion graft occlusion". Grading the severity of graft stenosis or classifying functional patency is best performed using the combination of duplex-derived velocity criteria, waveform analysis and resting ABI.

Essentials of Graft Surveillance

The need for graft surveillance varies with graft type, runoff, likelihood of residual postimplantation lesions, and whether limb pressures, e.g., pedal pulses, ABI, were normalized. In general, inflow procedures, such as aortofemoral, axillofemoral, femoral grafts do not require intensive postoperative surveillance. The incidence of technical errors and early failure is low (1-2%) as well as the concern for inadequate blood velocity as a mechanism for failure. Following inflow procedures, postimplantation lesions (occlusive or aneurysmal) typically develop at or near the femoral anastomosis and detection is possible by careful clinical evaluation that includes pulse palpation, auscultation for bruit, and serial measurement of ABI. By contrast, the hemodynamics and failure rate of infrainguinal bypass grafts mandate surveillance for a "low graft velocity state," a condition associated with residual/acquired graft stenosis and one which frequently precedes graft thrombosis.

Most patients who develop graft stenosis are asymptomatic, and a physical examination is insufficient to detect the subtle signs of the "hemodynamically failing, patent" graft. Less than one-quarter will have unequivocal evidence of graft stenosis on the basis of decreased pedal/graft pulse or recurrence of limb ischemia.[2,6,17,19] Screening of patients with angiography is not warranted because of the demographics of graft failure and the prohibitive risk and expense of serial angiographic evaluations. Although measurement of the resting ankle brachial systolic pressure index (ABI) is well established in diagnosis of arterial occlusive disease of the lower limb, this technique has low diagnostic sensitivity and specificity in detecting graft stenosis or predicting graft failure.[3,11,12] Barnes et al[11] found a decrease in ABI of >0.2 occurred with equal frequency in grafts that failed or remained patent. Multiple other investigators have also confirmed a positive predictive value in the range of 12-34% when ABI alone is used to predict graft thrombosis. In prospective studies using both duplex scanning and Doppler-derived ABI measurements, it was observed that graft thrombosis may occur despite normalization of ABI following surgery. An abnormal ABI in the perioperative period does not reliably identify grafts requiring revision.[7,9] Following infrainguinal saphenous vein bypass grafting, 20 (36%) of 56 graft stenoses were not apparent from serial measurements of resting ankle systolic pressure because of an insignificant change in the ABI (<0.15) or because the tibial arteries were incompressible, making pressure measurements unreliable. In contrast, all patients had abnormal duplex examinations based on changes in the magnitude and configuration of the graft velocity waveform. Graft stenosis was suspected when a low graft velocity state was detected and this finding then prompted complete duplex imaging of the arterial bypass. In 85% of patients examined, the location and severity of stenosis was ascertained. Two-thirds of the patients were asymptomatic despite a decrease in ABI to a mean of 0.62. Most investigators have observed that when patients develop recurrent symptoms of limb ischemia, frequently the graft has occluded. Similarly, while a decrease in ABI indicates a reduction in overall limb perfusion, resting ankle pressures do not always distinguish between functional normal, low-flow, or occluded grafts.

The combination of Doppler-derived ABIs and color-flow duplex imaging of the graft with duplex derived velocity determination can be used for monitoring vascular grafts. Color-flow imaging offers numerous advantages over conventional duplex scanning. Blood flow characteristics can be visualized over long segments, facilitating imaging both superficial and anatomically-positioned grafts, scanning the entire graft length including inflow vessels, anastomoses and runoff tract. Occlusive and aneurysmal lesions have "signature" color images thus eliminating the need for detailed center stream sampling for classifying severity. Accurate graft imaging does require the examiner be knowledgeable in a number of areas. (Table 3) At sites of stenosis, color-flow imaging typically demonstrates aliasing of the color map and a color-coded "flow jet," a hemodynamic characteristic of >50% diameter reduction lesions. Peak systolic velocities greater than 150-180 cm/sec, spectral broadening throughout the pulse cycle including reversed flow components in systole, and a velocity ratio greater than two are accepted duplex criteria of >50% diameter reduction stenosis. Grading stenosis severity and measurements of peak systolic velocity from normal graft segments must be performed using appropriate technique, including Doppler-corrected angles of 60 degrees or less. Instrumentation, scanning technique, and diagnostic

---

Table 3. Essentials of graft surveillance

Color duplex instrumentation
    Time-gain compensation
    Color coding algorithm
    Color maps

Pitfalls of color duplex imaging
    Aliasing
    Doppler angle correction

Arterial and bypass graft anatomy

Normal arterial and graft flow patterns

Measurement of duplex-derived blood flow velocities

Velocity spectra criteria for grading stenosis

Recognition of graft lesions
    Arteriovenous fistula
    Graft entrapment
    Anastomotic, vein graft aneurysms

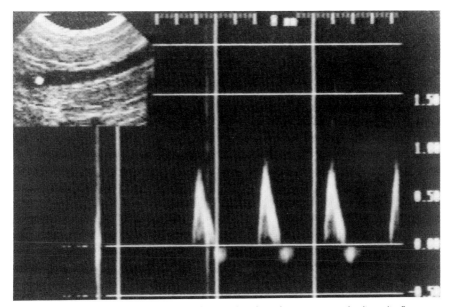

Figure 3. Duplex scan showing a PSV of 90 cm/sec but absent antegrade diastolic flow. An arteriogram showed a patent conduit but occluded outflow tract.

criteria are similar for monitoring both saphenous vein (in situ and reversed), autologous vein, prosthetic, and composite arterial bypasses.

SCANNING PROTOCOL AND ANATOMIC APPROACHES

Patients are placed in the supine position with the opposite hip shifted away from the leg being examined and the lower limb externally rotated. The knee is bent slightly. With the patient in this position, the arterial system from the aorta to the tibial arteries can be visualized. The examiner (vascular technologist or physician) should have available a complete description of the bypass graft procedure, the type and location of the conduit, sites of anastomoses, and any technical difficulties encountered at the primary operation. The bypass graft is visualized in the upper thigh and traced cephalad to the proximal anastomosis, typically the common femoral artery. The presence of triphasic waveform in the femoral artery correlates with a hemodynamically normal aortoiliac segment. In the presence of a patent graft, a pulsatility index greater than 4.0 also confirms the absence of inflow occlusive disease.[16] In questionable cases, the aortoiliac segment can be imaged directly for formation of plaque reducing the diameter of the lumen and abnormalities in flow pattern indicative of stenosis. Assessment of graft inflow, anastomotic sites and the graft conduit are mapped for structural abnormalities (stenosis, aneurysmal dilatation, intraluminal defect) and sites of flow disturbance. In situ vein bypasses lie superficial to the muscle fascia and are easily imaged throughout their length. When the saphenous vein is left in situ, the bypass conduit has a tapered configuration, with the segment with the largest diameter located in the thigh. Abrupt reductions in venous diameter typically occur at branch points and in duplicated venous segments. Reversed and prosthetic grafts commonly are placed through deep tunnels adjacent to the native vessels. Graft anastomoses to the below-knee popliteal artery are best imaged by using a posterior approach with the patient in a prone position. Anastomotic sites to the peroneal artery are the most difficult to examine because of their deeper location and their position behind the tibia. Distal graft stenosis typically are made in an end-to-side fashion to the native artery, thereby permitting blood to flow in both caudal and cephalad directions. When distal anastomotic sites cannot be imaged directly for analysis of the flow pattern, the functional resistance to flow (arterial impedance) of the anastomosis and outflow vessels can be assessed by the magnitude and configuration of the velocity waveform in the distal graft.

After the graft is imaged, center-stream velocity waveforms are recorded from several above and below-knee graft segments, where diameter does not vary and accurate assignment of the Doppler beam angle is possible. The magnitude and configuration of the velocity waveform are used for comparison with previous or subsequent studies obtained at the same recording site. It is not necessary to image the entire arterial system of the lower limb and the entire graft at each postoperative examination. Only grafts that develop a low peak systolic velocity less than 45 cm/sec or a decrease (more than 30 cm/sec) in blood-flow velocity require complete duplex mapping. When velocity measurements are used for predicting graft patency, the highest blood-flow velocity measured within the graft is used. For in situ bypasses, this corresponds to blood-flow velocity in the distal graft segment, whereas for reversed vein bypasses, the proximal graft segment should have the highest blood-flow velocity. Sites of flow disturbance are examined in detail to delineate the morphology of the lesion and to assess hemodynamic significance on the basis of changes in peak velocity and spectral content compared with normal proximal arterial segment.

Graft surveillance should be instituted in the operating room and should be repeated prior to discharge from the hospital with complete duplex mapping of the arterial bypass, measurement of graft blood-flow velocity and resting limb pressures. ABI, toe systolic pressure, wound edema, hematoma, and incisional tenderness may preclude detailed assessment of anastomotic sites in approximately 20% of patients for 2-3 weeks following surgery. After discharge from the hospital, graft surveillance should be repeated at six weeks, then at three-month intervals for two years, and every six months thereafter. This protocol appears adequate to detect the occasional rapid development of myointimal lesions that occur at valvular and anastomotic sites with moderate residual—<50% diameter reduction stenosis—flow/anatomic abnormalities. It appears that a normal duplex scan at three months is a good predictor for a low incidence of subsequent graft stenosis but further confirmation of this observation is required before the intervals of graft surveillance can be lengthened in this subgroup. In general, graft surveillance can be implemented by well-trained vascular laboratory personnel, and only when abnormalities are identified is a physician directed evaluation required.

CATEGORIES OF GRAFT STENOSIS

A localized increase in blood velocity and spectral broadening on duplex scanning identify the site of stenosis. On the basis of the velocity spectra of blood flow both distal and proximal to a stenotic vessel segment, severity can be classified into four disease categories: wall irregularity, less than 20%

diameter reduction (DR), 20% to 49% DR, 50% to 75% DR, and greater than 75% DR. In the two categories of greater than 50% DR stenosis, a pressure gradient exists across the lesion at the basal flow, and a reduction in ankle pressure can be measured. The finding of a lesion with the velocity spectrum of a stenosis greater than 50% has been uniformly associated with an angiographically detected lesion that warranted correction. The only exception to this observation has been in the identification of residual valve cusp(s) after in situ bypass during the perioperative period. Angiographically demonstrated lesions that show mild to moderate disruption in flow (stenosis less than 50%) on duplex scanning can be safely followed for progression, and when they are associated with a peak, systolic flow velocity greater than 45 cm/sec, graft failure has not occurred.

OUTCOME OF GRAFT SURVEILLANCE

A carefully conducted surveillance program should identify bypasses at risk for thrombosis, clarify the mechanism of graft failure, and reduce unexpected infrainguinal vein bypass failure to less than 2% per year. Following institution of a vein graft surveillance program at the Medical College of Wisconsin, a cumulative assisted primary patency of 96% at one year and 85% at five years was observed in patients undergoing in situ saphenous vein femorodistal bypass grafting. These results were superior to the three-year secondary patency of 47% observed when vein graft revision was undertaken on an acutely thrombosed in situ vein bypass. Common to all reports dealing with graft surveillance is the caveat stating the presence of symptomatic limb ischemia should not be a requisite criteria for graft revision. Since graft type, luminal diameter, configuration and runoff vary widely, the surveillance protocol should not be based on rigid criteria but rather designed to detect changes in baseline graft (peak systolic and end-diastolic velocity) and limb (ABI, toe systolic pressure) hemodynamics measured either at operation or in the perioperative period once a successful bypass is apparent. The combination allows detection of low velocity grafts, a hemodynamic state that commonly precedes graft failure (positive predictive value, 60-70%; negative predictive value, 95%). Interpreters of graft surveillance studies must remember the magnitude and configuration of the graft velocity waveform depends on several factors including: the recording site, the time interval after operation, and the outflow resistance of the runoff vessels. No single velocity criteria can be used to predict the likelihood of graft thrombosis. But in the setting of serial testing, we have observed an increased failure rate, especially for prosthetic grafts, when the maximum (measured from the smallest diameter but normal graft segment) graft systolic velocity was less than 40 cm/sec and no forward diastolic forward flow was present.

The decision of when to recommend graft revision has not been clearly defined, except when patients have recurrent symptoms of claudication or have developed ischemic lesions. The scenario of recurrent limb ischemia was observed in only one-third of our patients despite conclusive vascular laboratory studies for a "hemodynamically failing" bypass graft.

REFERENCES

1. Sladen JD, Gilmour JL. Vein graft stenosis: characteristics and effect of treatment. Am J Surg 1981; 141:549-551.

2. Turnipseed WD, Acher CW. Postoperative surveillance: an effective means of detecting correctable lesions that threaten graft patency, Arch Surg 1985;120:324-326.

3. Bandyk DF, Cato RF, Towne JB. A low flow velocity predicts failure of femoropopliteal and femorotibial bypass. Surgery 1985; 98:799-802.

4. Green RM, McNamara L, Ouriel K, Deweese JA. Comparison of infrainguinal graft surveillance techniques. J Vasc Surg 1990; 11:207-215.

5. Bandyk DF, Schmitt DD, Seabrook GR, Adams MB, Towne JB. Monitoring functional patency of in situ saphenous vein bypasses: The impact of a surveillance protocol and elective revision. J Vasc Surg 1989; 9:284-296.

6. Sladen JG, Reid JDS, Cooperberg PL. Color flow duplex screening of infrainguinal grafts combining low- and high-velocity criteria. Am J Surg 1989; 158:107-112.

7. Mills JL, Harris EJ, Taylor LM, Beckett WC. The importance of routine surveillance of distal bypass grafts with duplex scanning: A study of 379 reversed vein grafts. J Vasc Surg 1990; 12:379-389.

8. Londrey GL, Hodgson KJ, Spadone DP, Ramsey DE, Barkmeier LD, Sumner DS. Initial experience with color-flow duplex scanning of infrainguinal bypass grafts. J Vasc Surg 1990; 12:284-290.

9. Disselhoff B, Buth J, Jakimowicz J. Early detection of stenosis of femoro-distal grafts. A surveillance study using color-duplex scanning. Eur J Vasc Surg 1989; 3:43

10. Buth J, Disselhoff B, Sommeling C, Stam L. Color-flow duplex criteria for grading stenosis in infrainguinal vein grafts. J Vasc Surg 1991; 14:716-728.

11. Barnes RW, Thompson BW, MacDonald CM et al. Serial noninvasive studies do not herald postoperative failure of femoropopliteal or femorotibial bypass grafts. Ann Surg 1989; 210:486-494.

12. Bandyk DF, Sumna DS, Thiele BL, Yao JST. Clinical research trials using noninvasive vascular testing. J Vasc Surg 1992; 15:897-901.

13. Grigg MJ, Nicolaides AN, Wolfe JHN. Femorodistal vein graft stenoses. Br J Surg 1988; 75:737-740.

14. Moody AP, Gould DA, Harris PL. Vein graft surveillance improves patency in femoropoliteal bypass. Eur J Vasc Surg 1990; 4:117-121.

15. Idu MM, Blankenstein JD, de Gier P, Truyen E, Buth J. Impact of a color-flow duplex surveillance program on infrainguinal vein graft patency. A five-year experience. (Abstract) J Vasc Surg 1992;

16. Mattos MA, van Bemmelen PS, Hodgson KJ, Ramsey DE, Barkmeier LD, Sumner DS. Does correction of stenoses identified with color duplex scanning improve infrainguinal graft patency? (Abstract) J Vasc Surg 1992; 17:54-64.

17. Donaldson MC, Mannick JA, Whittemore AD. Causes of primary graft failure after in situ saphenous vein bypass grafting. J Vasc Surg 1992; 15:113-120.

18. Bergamini TM, Towne JB, Bandyk DF, Seabrook GR, Schmitt DD. Experience with in situ saphenous vein bypasses during 1981 to 1989.

Determinant factors of long-term patency. J Vasc Surg 1991; 13:137-149.

19. Sauvage LR, Walker MW, Berger KG et al. Current arterial prostheses, Arch Surg 1979; 114:687-692.

20. Bandyk DF, Seabrook GR, Moldenhauer P, Lavin J, Edwards J, Cato R, Towne JB. Hemodynamics of vein graft stenosis. J Vasc Surg 1988; 8:688-695.

21. Bandyk DF, Kaebnick, Bergamini TM et al. Hemodynamics of in situ saphenous vein arterial bypass. Arch Surg 123:477, 1988.

22. Belkin M, Mackey WC, McLaughlin R, Humphrey SE, O'Donnell TF. The variation in vein graft flow velocity with luminal diameter and outflow level. J Vasc Surg 1992; 15:991-999.

CHAPTER 6

SURVEILLANCE OF LOWER EXTREMITY VEIN GRAFTS

Jaap Buth

THE RATIONALE FOR VEIN GRAFT SURVEILLANCE

The causes of failure of lower extremity vein grafts following the perioperative period can be separated into those that are amenable to surgical or endovascular intervention and those that are not. Failure due to diffuse disease in the run off vessels and hypercoagulability belong to the latter group and only medical therapy, such as anticoagulation, may be beneficial in these situations. Stenotic lesions in the graft and the anastomotic areas may be treated invasively. In the first three months these are usually technical problems. After three months these abnormalities are most frequently caused by myointimal hyperplasia and are responsible for most graft failures within the first postoperative year; 65-75% of all graft failures occur within the first year.[1] Progression of atherosclerotic lesions as a cause of graft thrombosis is generally seen after the first year when the annual graft attrition rate becomes approximately 2-3%.

As the long-term patency of grafts following thrombectomy or thrombolysis ranges from 19 to 28%, follow-up of patients with infrainguinal vein grafts should be directed towards the identification of the failing graft.[2,3] At this stage relatively minor revisions can often avert graft failure. It has been shown that the secondary patency of electively revised grafts is comparable with the primary patency in bypasses without stenoses.[4]

Only one-third of hemodynamically significant graft stenoses are diagnosed by the return of ischemic symptoms or decreased pulses at physical examination. In contrast, it has been shown that periodic surveillance using intravenous digital subtraction angiography (IV-DSA) or noninvasive methods, such as duplex, is effective in identifying graft stenosis. Using these methods the incidence of stenotic lesions has been found to be up to 25-30% of vein grafts in the first year.[5-11] The majority of stenoses develop within the first postoperative year. Consequently, although in a recent report Sanchez et

Reprinted by permission from the European Journal of Vascular Surgery.

al[12] advocate indefinite postoperative surveillance, most investigators favor restriction to a 12-month period.

Which bypasses should be systematically followed? There is no significant difference between the incidence of myointimal hyperplasia or valve cusp fibrosis in in situ and reversed vein grafts [13] and it has been shown experimentally that endothelial damage in vein grafts can be induced by the changed hemodynamic circumstances of arterialization.[14]

This does not, however, explain the localized nature of stenotic graft lesions. Moody et al did not find a correlation between developing stenoses and clamp sites in grafts, clipped tributary veins, residual valve cusps or venotomy sites.[15] However, endothelial desquamation by intraluminal instrumentation or irrigation with nonphysiological solutions is a likely factor in that it initiates local platelet deposition which is a precursor of stenosis formation. Whether pre-existing vein wall fibrosis is a common causal factor is not known.

Data on surveillance of PTFE bypasses are scarce. Stenosis formation because of a compliance mismatch and local flow disturbance at the hood of the proximal or distal anastomosis does occur. However, in the study of Taylor et al only 7% of PTFE prostheses developed stenotic lesions as compared with 19% of vein grafts.[16] At the present time it is uncertain whether the higher failure rate of prosthetic infrainguinal bypasses can be decreased by periodic noninvasive assessment.

Correction of high-grade stenotic lesions may improve long-term graft patency rates by approximately 15%.[7,17] For this reason in recent years surveillance programs of femoro-distal vein grafts using noninvasive methods have been started in many institutions. The purpose of this review is to discuss diagnostic methods, criteria for stenosis and recommendations for intervention that are currently applied for vein graft surveillance.

THE VALUE OF ANKLE BLOOD PRESSURE MEASUREMENTS IN THE DETECTION OF GRAFT STENOSES

Measurement of ABI is widely used for the assessment of the integrity of native arteries and reconstructed segments. This test has been used extensively as an indicator of significant stenoses in grafts or adjacent inflow and run-off arteries.[6,8,19] In an earlier series of 77 grafts from our institution which were screened with ABI, color flow duplex and IV-DSA, 13 severe grafts or anastomotic stenoses were identified during the follow-up period.[20] A decrease in the ABI of more than 0.15 was considered to indicate a significant obstruction. In this study only 31% of significant graft stenoses could be diagnosed using this criterion. Other investigators have found that in 50-80% of cases significant stenoses were missed by serial determination of ABI[21-23] (and A.L. Laborde et al, unpublished data). The potential of the interval drop of the resting ABI in identifying impending graft failure as well as the presence of a significant stenoses has been investigated at different threshold values. Respective decreases of 0.20, 0.15 and 0.10 were evaluated, but no accurate indicator has been found from serial ABI investigations.[20,21,23,24-26] The narrow diagnostic range of ABI is its major limitation for the identification of graft stenosis.

Values of less than 0.15 fall within the biological and measurement variations of the test, while values greater than 0.20 are often associated with an occluded graft rather than with a failing bypass. This may be explained by the tendency of pressures to fall precipitously once the graft diameter is critically reduced. As the interval between measurements is usually three months, there is a remote chance that progression to the point of graft thrombosis will be picked up.

Some studies have suggested that ABI combined with ankle pressure measurements post-exercise (ABPE) can improve diagnostic sensitivity [27] but in our experience graft stenoses are often missed by the ABPE measurements as well. Another drawback of this test is that the typically older patient population cannot often perform the treadmill exercise adequately. It may be possible to overcome this by a reactive hyperemia test as is used for the assessment of peripheral arterial disease.[28]

Other aspects limit the value of ankle pressures for the identification of impending graft failure. Pressures cannot be determined in at least 20% of diabetic patients due to incompressible vessels and very distal bypasses preclude the identification of graft lesions beyond the ankle level. Furthermore, a decrease in ABI or ABPE often coincides with the return of symptoms, rendering the measurements superfluous in these cases.

Despite its limited diagnostic value in detecting stenotic lesions, the measurement of ankle blood pressures will undoubtedly remain part of the follow-up examination. This method is suitable for documenting graft occlusion when foot pulses are not palpable. In addition ABI is used by some investigators to supplement a duplex surveillance protocol; grafts with evidence of stenoses are being followed at frequent intervals until symptoms occur or a drop in ABI develops. [26,29]

ANGIOGRAPHY AS A FOLLOW-UP TOOL

The report by Szilagyi et al in 1973 emphasizing the concept that intrinsic lesions develop within vein grafts and constitute a threat to patency, was based on findings of an arteriographic follow-up.[5] In addition these investigators examined recovered graft material histopathologically. Angiography provides fine anatomical detail and thus enabled Szilagyi to discriminate six types of structural changes in grafts: intimal thickening, atherosclerosis, fiberotic valve, suture line stenosis, fiberotic (traumatic) stenosis and aneurysmal dilation. Conventional arteriography, however, is cumbersome, not completely without risk, and too expensive to be used for routine follow-up screening.

Consequently, in later studies its use has been confined to determining the localization and severity of a stenotic lesion after its presence had been suspected because of clinical symptoms or a decrease in ankle pressure. Intraoperative arteriography has been employed to identify the cause of graft failure after thrombectomy.[2,8] Moody et al., Wolfe et al and Turnipseed et al have all employed IV-DSA to detect failing but patent grafts.[11,21,30] However, because of a lack of spatial resolution, IV-DSA does not always allow adequate visualization of the entire bypass or an accurate assessment of diameter reduction. The hazards of repeated radiation, in addition to the high costs of angiography, make this technique inappropriate as a serial diagnostic procedure.

Both intravenous and intra-arterial DSA have been used as "gold standards" to establish criteria for the noninvasive grading of lesions as well as management protocols. Furthermore, angiographic confirmation is usually requested before corrective intervention is contemplated. One may assume that once the reliability of noninvasive duplex is settled the need for angiography will diminish and a substantial proportion of graft revisions will be undertaken without prior angiography.

DUPLEX AND COLOR FLOW DUPLEX SURVEILLANCE OF VEIN GRAFTS

Duplex scanning has been used for several years in diagnosing and grading carotid and peripheral arterial disease as well as venous disorders. The relatively late application of duplex scanning as a screening method is due to several factors. First, the assumption that ankle pressure measurements were accurate in indicating impending graft failure. Although Berkowitz and coworkers [31] were able to detect graft stenoses in as many as 21 of the grafts using standard follow-up techniques, a number of recent comparative studies have clearly demonstrated that duplex scanning is a superior method.[16,20,22,25,32,33] Furthermore, moderate graft stenoses (30-50% diameter reduction) may also be diagnosed by duplex scanning. Progression of lesions can be followed and timely interventions be planned depending on the assessed risk of graft thrombosis.

A drawback of conventional grey-scale duplex is the time involved in peripheral graft examination; especially when high-velocity criteria are used, several pulsed Doppler velocity samplings along the entire length of the graft are required to search for stenotic lesions. The use of color flow duplex is less cumbersome and this method appears particularly suited to examining peripheral blood vessels and infrainguinal bypasses.[20,34-36] (See also Laborde et al, unpublished data.) Stenotic segments can be identified by locally increased peak velocities and poststenotic turbulence characterized by color-coded forward and reversed flow. The diameter changes are measured and recorded in longitudinal and transverse projections. Quantitative pulsed Doppler velocity measurements can be performed as in conventional duplex scanning. In Figure 1 parameters as used in our laboratory are summarized. The advent of the in situ graft has brought some additional advantages for the use of duplex scanning. In anatomically routed reversed vein grafts, segments in the distal thigh were often difficult to investigate.

The costs of repetitive duplex scanning may have discouraged its application for graft surveillance programs. Wolfe and coworkers calculated that if limb loss was prevented in only 2% of patients a duplex surveillance program would be cost-effective for health-care insurance companies.[37] While their calculations may now have to be adjusted to the more frequent use of color flow duplex scanners, which are more expensive but less time consuming, the economic advantages of the prevention of amputations can easily be demonstrated.

In Table 1 the criteria and potential of several duplex parameters for the identification of failing grafts or stenotic lesions are compared. Low-velocity and high-velocity duplex criteria can be discriminated. The former criterion only requires measurement of the peak systolic velocity (PSV) at some fixed points of the anastomotic areas and at mid-graft level and is therefore easier to use when a conventional duplex scanner is involved. We have found that although a low PSV-graft usually indicated a high grade stenosis (high positive predictive value) the actual proportion of severe lesions with a positive test is small (low sensitivity).[35] This observation is in accord with

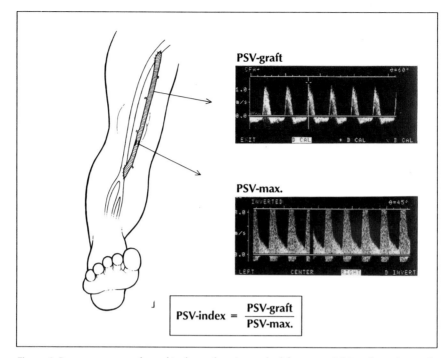

Figure 1. Parameters as evaluated in the authors' vascular laboratory: PSV-graft, peak systolic velocity measured at the normal midthigh graft; PSV-max, peak systolic velocity measured at the stenosis or, in normal in situ bypasses, at the below knee graft; PSV-index, ratio of the PSV-graft and PSV-max; EDV, end-diastolic velocity at the stenosis, or in normal bypasses at the below-knee graft. The PSV-index is the reciprocal value of the V2/V1 ratio d. (See Tables 1 and 2.) In normal grafts the PSV-index is close to 1.0, while stenotic bypasses are characterized by lower values. (Reproduced with permission from the Journal of Vascular Surgery)

Table 1. Duplex parameters and criteria for stenotic lesions in femorodistal vein grafts and adjacent arteries

Parameters	Criteria	Potential
Low velocity PSV graft	< 45 cms	*Indicates:* →Impending graft failure →Inflow and runoff disease
High velocity V1/V2 ratio*	>1.5 ↓	*Discriminates:* →All stenoses from normal grafts
PSV-index∞	< 0.65	→Moderate stenoses from normal graft
EDV	>20 cms	→Severe stenoses from moderate stenoses
Color flow image	Direct measurement % diameter reduction	*Discriminates:* →mild stenosis from moderate stenosis

* Stenosis/normal graft
∞ Normal graft/stenosis
For abbreviations, see footnotes to Figure 1.

Table 2. Reported series with different criteria used for duplex or color-flow duplex identification of graft stenoses

Source	Duplex criteria	No. of grafts	Stenoses No.	Stenoses %	Electively revised patency grafts No.	%	Thrombosed grafts No.	%	Secondary patency %
Duplex									
Bandyk et al (1987)	PSV-graft<45 cms⁻¹	192	33	17	29	15	21	11	89 (3 years)
McShane et al (1987)	PSV shift	74	25	34	8	11	9	12	Not reported
Grigg et al (1988)*	V2/V1>1.5	80	19	24	5	6	7	9	Not reported
Green et al (1990)	PSV-graft<40 cms⁻¹ PSV-max >120 cms⁻¹	177	Not reported		20	11	18	10	80 (5 years)
Mills et al (1990),	PSV changes between visits (50%) PSV-graft <45 cms⁻¹ Vs/V1 >1.5	379	48	13	48	13	20	5	Not reported
Taylor et al (1990)*	Distal flow < 25 ml min⁻¹	412	66	16	30	7	Not reported for total series		Not reported
Chang et al (1990)	Hyperemic/resting flow <2.5 Vein graft size <3 mm PSV-graft <45 cms⁻¹								
Color flow duplex									
Disselhoff et al (1989)	V2/V1 >1.3	77	18	23†	13	17	Not reported		70 (2 years)
Sladen et al (1989)	V2/V1 >2 PSV-max >300 cms⁻¹ PSV-graft <45 cms⁻¹	114	39	34†	Not reported		Not reported		Not reported
Londrey et al (1990)	V2/B1 >2	76	15	20	5	7	6	8	Not reported
Buth et al (1991)	PSV-index <0.65 PSV-graft <45 cms⁻¹ Color-flow image %DR	115	43	37†	31	27	11	10	91 (2 years‡)
Corson et al (unpublished data)	EDV >20 cms⁻¹ V2/V1 >3 PSV-graft <45 cms⁻¹	124	38	31†	30	24	9	7	87 (3 years)

For abbreviations see footnote to Figure 1.　　　* Duplex or IV-DSA used for surveillance.　　　† Stenoses <50% diameter reduction included.　　　‡ First month failures not considered.

Laborde et al (Laborde et al, unpublished data). Nevertheless a low PSV-graft is associated with a high incidence of graft occlusion during follow-up.[39] Graft stenoses may not however account entirely for this, as low PSV-graft values are frequently caused by run-off or inflow disease.[33,34,36]

In duplex scanning graft volume flow has evolved as an unsatisfactory indicator stenosis. This measurement was found to be unreproducible within the graft itself from one observer to another and from one visit to the next one since cardiac output and peripheral resistance affect blood flow.[40] A ratio of hyperemic blood flow/resting blood flow of less than 2.5 was found to be significantly correlated with bypass compromise.[38] However the predictive value of this test is too limited for it to be used as an indicator for confirmative angiography.

Color flow duplex, as described above, permits efficient tracing of the entire graft and is therefore more suitable with high-velocity criteria that represent the change in Doppler shift between normal and stenotic graft segments. A proportional increase of the PSV at a stenosis compared with a normal arterial segment was first described as an indicator for disease in native arteries by Jager et al.[41] Grigg et al and Bandyk have used this relative increase of flow velocity to study vein grafts.[9,29]

Grigg uses a "V2/V2-ratio" (stenosis/normal graft peak systolic velocities) and calculated that a ratio of 1.5 discriminated normal grafts accurately from those with a mild to moderate stenosis. This increase is equivalent to a PSV-index of below 0.65, as we have been using. We found this criterion accurate for the identification of a graft stenosis of 50% or greater diameter reduction (DR) with a sensitivity of 89% and a specificity of 92%. We chose to use an index with a normal value of approximately 1.0 and lower values indicating stenosis.

Increase of the end-diastolic velocity (EDV) of greater than 20 cm has in our hands provided a good indicator of stenoses greater than 69% (sensitivity 91%, specificity 100%). Direct measurements of diameter reduction by color flow imaging appeared a reliable parameter for the discrimination of mild and moderate stenoses (>30% DR and >50% DR, respectively) from normal grafts. On the basis of these parameters it is possible to grade a stenotic lesion and assess how far a graft is compromised.

Table 2 summarizes the observations from a number of reports and the duplex criteria used. The frequency of graft stenosis varies from 16 to 37% depending on whether low- or high-velocity criteria are used and stenoses less than 50% diameter reduction are taken into account. The frequency of graft revision varied in series from 7 to 21% and this appears to be related to the rate of identification of stenotic lesions. Secondary patency rates are often not reported, which renders comparison difficult. The rate of thrombosed grafts without any reintervention appears low for all series suggesting an overall beneficial effect of graft surveillance.

RESULTS OF GRAFT REVISION AND RECOMMENDATIONS FOR MANAGEMENT OF IDENTIFIED GRAFT LESIONS

Repair of vein graft stenoses has been performed successfully for more than two decades.[42,43] Patch angioplasty, excision of stenotic segments with direct repair, segmental graft placement or (jump) extension grafts are the most common operative methods for revision. The results of percutaneous transluminal angioplasty (PTA) are less durable than those of surgical revision, as combined recurrence and failure rates of 33-50% are seen,[44-48] and a poor result can be expected especially when lesions longer than 1 cm are involved.

Historical controls, literature data or nonrandomized control groups have been used for comparisons with the patencies obtained in the duplex surveillance groups.[17,49] In the study by Moody et al a significantly higher patency rate was observed in the study group as compared with nonscreened grafts.[17] In 1989 Bandyk reported comparable four-year patency rates in grafts without a stenotic lesion and grafts with revised stenoses.[10] In a retrospective study from our department the patency of 33 stenotic but revised grafts compared favorably with the patency in 15 stenotic grafts that had not undergone a revisional procedure for various reasons. The secondary three-year patency in revised grafts was 93% as opposed to 53% in nonrevised grafts.[50] Thus there seems little disagreement between investigators that the tendency for graft failure is high in the presence of noncorrected stenosis. Stenotic lesions, especially severe ones, do not tolerate delay in treatment. In contrast, grafts with mild to moderate stenosis (<50% DR) do not appear to be at great risk of occlusion and remain stable for long periods.

CONCLUSION

In spite of the data mentioned above there is no complete consensus about the benefit of searching out and repairing early graft lesions.[25] The question of whether duplex surveillance is a prerequisite for optimal patient care following infrainguinal bypass grafting can only be answered after a randomized study comparing groups with and without intervention of these lesions has been accomplished.

Which approach should be recommended meanwhile? An active search for stenotic lesions following bypass grafting is justified by the results as currently reported by different investigators. As most stenoses begin early after the operation, duplex screening should start no later than the sixth postoperative week. Subsequent follow-up studies should be performed at 3, 6, 9 and 12 months. If within the first postoperative year no stenosis has developed, longer duplex screening would have a low yield and may not be cost effective. Grafts with treated stenoses should be followed for at least another year as recurrences can be expected in about one out of four grafts.[10,16,32]

Mapping and calculation of percentage stenosis by duplex is feasible. We currently recommend an angiographic study when a stenosis of 50% or greater is suspected. Graft revision may be considered when a significant stenosis is confirmed by angiography. When a stenosis of greater than 70% is found, corrective intervention of the lesion is urgently needed. One may forgo angiography in these cases if a good duplex study of the entire infrainguinal bypass has been obtained.

REFERENCES

1. Brewster DC, LaSalle AJ, Robison JG, Darling RC. Femoropopliteal graft failures. Clinical consequences and success of secondary reconstructions. Arch Surg 1983; 118: 1043-1047.
2. Cohen JR, Mannick JA, Couch NP, Whittemore AD. Recognition and management of impending vein-graft failure. Importance for long-terrn patency. Arch Surg 1986; 121: 758-759.

3. Belkin M, Donaldson MC, Whittemore AD et al. Observations of the use of thrombolytic agents for thrombotic occlusions of infrainguinal vein grafts. J Vasc Surg 1990; 11: 289-296.

4. Bandyk DF, Schmitt DD, Seabrook GR, Adams MB, Towne JB. Monitoring functional patency of in situ saphenous vein bypasses: The impact of a surveillance protocol and elective revision. J Vasc Surg 1989; 9: 286-296.

5. Szilagy DE, Eliot JP, Haglesman JH, Smith RF, Sallolmo CA. Biological fate of autologous vein implants as arterial substitutes. Ann Surg 1973; 178: 232-246.

6. Berkowitz H, Hobbs CH, Roberts B, Friedman D, Oleaga J, Ring E. Value of routine vascular laboratory studies to identify vein graft stenoses. Surgery 1981; 90: 971-979.

7. Sladen JG, Gilmour JL. Vein graft stenosis: Characteristics and effect of treatment. Am J Surg 1981; 41: 549-553.

8. Whittemore AD, Clowes AW, Couch NP, Mannick JA. Secondary femoropopliteal reconstruction. Ann Surg 1981;193: 35-42

9. Grigg MJ, Nicolaides AN, Wolfe JHN. Femorodistal vein bypass graft stenosis. Br J Surg 1988; 75: 737-740.

10. Leopold PW, Shandal AA, Kay C et al. Duplex ultrasound: Its role in the noninvasive follow-up of the in situ saphenous vein bypass. J Vasc Technol 1987;11: 183-186.

11. Moody P, DeCossart LM, Douglas HM, Harris PL. Asymptomatic strictures in femoropopliteal vein grafts. Eur J Vasc Surg 1989; 3: 389-392.

12. Sanchez LA, Gupta SK, Veith FJ et al. A ten-year experience with one hundred fifty failing or threatened vein and polyetrafluoroethylene arterial bypass grafts. J Vasc Surg 1991; 14: 729-738.

13. Harris PL, DeCossart LM, Moody P, Douglas H. How can we detect and manage fibrous strictures within new grafts? Are these more problematic with reversed than in situ bypass? In: Greenhaugh RM, Jamieson CW, Nicolaides AN, eds. Limb Salvage and Amputation for Vascular Disease. London: W.B. Saunders, 1988: 221-231.

14. Buch HL, Jabukowski JA, Curl R, Deykin D, Nasbeth, DC. .The natural history of endothelial structure and function in arterialized vein grafts. J Vasc Surg 1986; 3: 204-215.

15. Moody, P, Gould DA, Harris PL. Vein graft screening: A prospective study of etiological factors. (Abstr.) Br J Surg 1991; 78: 371.

16. Taylor PR, Wolfe JHN, Tyrrell MR, Mansfield AO, Nicolaides AN, Houston RN. Graft stenosis: Justification for one-year surveillance. Br J Surg 1990; 77:1125-1128.

17. Moody P, Gould DA, Harris PL. Vein graft surveillance improves patency in femoropopliteal bypass. Eur J Vasc Surg 1990; 4: 117-121.

18. Sumner DS, Standness DE. Hemodynamic studies before and after extended bypass grafts to the tibial and peroneal arteries. Surgery 1979; 86: 442-452.

19. O'Mara CS, Flinn WR, Johnson ND, Bergan JJ, Yao JST. Recognition and surgical management of patent but hemodynamically failed arterial grafts. Ann Surg 1981; 193: 467-476.

20. Disselhoff B, Buth J, Jakimowicz J. Early detection of stenosis of femoro-

distal grafts. A surveillance study using color duplex scanning. Eur J Vasc Surg 1989; 3: 43-18.

21. Wolfe JHN, Thomas ML, Jamieson CW, Browse NL, Burnland KG, Rutt, DL. Early diagnosis of femorodistal graft stenosis. Br J Surg 1987; 74: 268-270.

22. McShane MD, Gazzard VM, Clifford PC, Humphries KN, Webster JHH, Chant ADB. Duplex ultrasound monitoring arterial grafts: prospective evaluation in conjunction with ankle pressure indices after femorodistal bypass. Eur J Vasc Surg 1987; 1: 385-390.

23. Mills JL, Harris JE, Taylor LM, Beckett WC, Porter JM. The Importance of routine surveillance of distal bypass grafts with duplex scanning: a study of 379 reversed vein grafts. J Vasc Surg 1990; 12:379-389.

24. Bandyk DF, Seabrook GR, Mildenhauer P et al. Hemodynamics of vein graft stensosis. J Vasc Surg 1988; 8:688-695.

25. Barnes RW, Thompson BW, MacDonald CM et al. Serial noninvasive studies do not herald postoperative failure of femoropopliteal or femorotibial bypass grafts. Ann Surg 1989; 210: 486-494.

26. Green RM, McNamara J, Ouriel K, DeWeese JA. Comparison of infrainguinal graft surveillance techniques. J Vasc Surg 1990; 11: 207-215.

27. Brennan JA, Walsh AKM, Beard JD, Bolia AA, Bell PRF. The role of simple noninvasive testing in infrainguinal vein graft surveillance. Eur J Vasc Surg 1991; 5: 13-17.

28. Verhagen PF, DeJong TJ, Van Vronnhoven THJ. Ankle pressure changes during reactive hyperemia in peripheral arterial disease. Vasa 1983; 12: 29-34.

29. Bandyk DF. Postoperative surveillance of infrainguinal bypass. Surg Clin North Am 1990; 70: 71-85.

30. Turnipseed WD, Acher CW. Postoperative surveillance. An effective means of detecting correctable lesions that threaten graft patency. Arch Surg 1985;120: 324-328.

31. Berkowitz HD, Greenstein S, Barker CF, Perloff LJ. Late failure of reversed vein bypass grafts. Ann Surg 1989; 210: 782-786.

32. Grigg MJ, Nicolaides AN, Wolfe JHN. Detection and grading of femorodistal vein gratt stenoses: Duplex measurements with angiography, J Vasc Surg 1988: 8: 661-666.

33. Sladen JG, Reid JDS, Cooperberg PL et al. Color flow duplex screening of infrainguinal gratts combining low and high-velocity criteria. Am J Surg 1989; 158: 112.

34. Londrey GL, Hodgson KJ, Spadone DP, Ramsey DE, Barkmeier LD, Sumner DS. Initial experience with color-flow duplex scanning of infrainguinal bypass grafts. J Vasc Surg 1990; 12: 284- 90.

35. Buth J, Disselhoff B, Sommeling C, Stam L. Color-flow duplex criteria for grading stenosis in infrainguinal vein grafts. J Vasc Surg 1991; 14: 716-728.

36. Cosman P, Salles-Cunha S, Andros G. Duplex ultrasonography of infrainguinal bypass grafts. J Vasc Technol 1989;13:127

37. Wolfe JHN, Taylor PR, Cheshire NJ. Graft surveillance. A biased overview. In: Greenhalgh RM, Holier LM, ed. The Maintenance of Arterial Reconstruction. London: W.B. Saunders, 1991: 119-127.

38. Chang BB, Leather RP, Kaufman JL, Kupinsky AM, Leopold PW, Shah DM. Hemodynamic characteristics of failing infrainguinal in situ bypass. J Vasc Surg 1990:12: 597-600.

39. Bandyk DF, Cato RF, Towne JB. A low-flow velocity predicts failure of femoro-popliteal and femorotibial bypass grafts. Surgery 1985; 98: 799-809.

40. Grigg MF, Wolfe JHN, Tovar A, Nicolaides AN. The reliability of duplex derived hemodynamic measurement in assessment of femorodistal grafts. Eur J Vasc Surg 1988; 2: 177-181.

41. Jager KA, Phillips DJ, Martin RL et al. Noninvasive mapping of lower limb arterial lesions. Ultrasound Med Bio 1985; 11: 515-521.

42. Breslau RC, DeWeese JA. Successful endophlebectomy of autogenous venous bypass grafts. Ann Surg 1965; 162: 251-254.

43. McNamara RC, Darling RC, Linton RR. Segmental stenosis of saphenous vein autografts: Preventable cause of late occlusion in arterial reconstruction. N Engl J Med 1967; 277: 290-292.

44. Bandyk DF, Bergamini TM, Towne JB, Schmitt DD, Seabrook GR. Durability of vein graft revision: The outcome of secondary procedures. J Vasc Surg 1991; 13: 200-210.

45. Harris PL, Moody AP. The management of vein bypass strictures. In: The Maintenance of Arterial Reconstruction. London: W.B.Saunders. 1991: 169-179.

46. Thompson JF, McShane MD, Clifford PC, Gazzard V, Webster JH, Chant AB. Intervention for graft stenoses: The role of surgery and transluminal angioplasty. Br J Surg 1988; 76: 1017.

47. Perler BA, Osterman FA, Mitchell SE, Burdick JF, Williams GM. Balloon dilatation versus surgical revision of infrainguinal autogenous vein graft stenosis long-term follow-up. J Cardiovasc Surg 1990; 14: 340-345.

48. Whittemore AD, Donaldson MC, Polak JF, Mannick JA. Limitations of balloon angioplasty for vein graft stenosis. J Vasc Surg 1991; 14: 340-345.

49. Bandyk DF, Keabnick HW, Stewart GW, Towne JB. Durability of the in situ saphenous vein arterial bypass: A comparison of primary and secondary patency. J Vasc Surg 1987; 5: 256-268.

50. Buth J, Disselhoff B, Truyen E, Stam L. Can color duplex surveillance of femorodistal vein bypasses result in reduction of graft failures. In: Greenhalgh RM, Hollier LM, eds. The Maintenance of Arterial Reconstruction. London: W.B. Saunders 1991; 105-117.

CHAPTER 7

REMOTE MONITORING OF GRAFT FUNCTION

Sushil K. Gupta
Frank J. Veith

The previous chapters have clearly demonstrated that a steady decline with time in patency of vascular grafts occurs and therefore a protocol of postoperative surveillance to identify grafts at risk of thrombosis is mandatory. Detection of the stenotic lesions before the graft thromboses is important because correction of these lesions requires relatively simple procedures and results in better patency rates.[1-4] In comparison, the thrombosed grafts require more complex procedures and results are poor.[2]

As shown in the earlier chapter by Green et al, the postoperative surveillance using Ankle Pressure Gradient (APG) and pulse volume recording is not always effective. A considerable number of patients develop thrombosis in the intervening period between the procedure and the noninvasive examination. Duplex ultrasound examinations are a better tool for detecting prethombosis but these exams are time-consuming, expensive and often ineffective because graft failure may still occur without premonitory symptoms or signs in the interval between examinations.

In this chapter, we present results using an implantable piezoelectric polymer graft monitoring device. Piezoelectric transducers can convert the mechanical motion of graft pulsation to an electrical signal that may be quantified and monitored periodically. This device allows continuous, on-line monitoring of graft function and may result in improved detection of failing grafts.

MATERIAL AND METHODS

PIEZOELECTRIC SENSORS

Piezoelectric film is available in sheets of polyvinylident fluoride (PVF2) of varying thicknesses ranging from 6 μm to 110 μm and is metallized on one or both surfaces with different metals (nickel, aluminum, and silver, among

Reprinted by permission from the American Journal of Surgery.

others) depending on the application (Pennwalt, Valley Forge, PA). For the purposes of these experiments, we made our sensors from a 28 μm thick film metallized on both surfaces with silver ink in a rectangle measuring 12 cm x 0.5 cm. This strip was then folded over in the center and the two inside metallic surfaces were bonded to an electrode made of copper tape; a silver-containing epoxy was used for the bonding. The sensors were insulated on the outside by bonding a 5 μm mylar film with an insulating epoxy. These sensors were then wrapped around a 6 mm polytetrafluorethylene (PTFE) graft in a spiral manner and bonded to the outer surface of the graft with silicone epoxy.

In Vitro Testing

To evaluate the response of the piezoelectric vascular graft sensor (PGS) in vitro, a pulsatile pump, which was connected to tubing 5/8 inches in diameter, was used in a configuration simulating an arterial tree containing multiple branches. A 6 mm PTFE graft with a PGS wrapped around it was then attached in series in the middle of one of the arterial branches. The pulsatile pump was primed with saline and calibrated to a pulsatile flow of 300 ml/minute. The output from the PGS was fed into a high output impedence amplifier.

In Vivo Testing

Ten 6 mm PTFE grafts containing PGSs were connected end-to-end between the external iliac and the common femoral arteries bilaterally in five anesthetized dogs. An electromagnetic flow meter was placed around the common femoral artery just beyond the distal anastomosis of the PTFE graft. An intraluminal pressure transducer was added via a needle inserted in the PTFE graft at the level of the PGS. The signals from all three sources were fed into a DATAQ A/D acquisition board placed in an IBM-ST computer, and CODAS data acquisition software was used to acquire real time data at a frequency of 200 Hz. All data were graphically displayed on a computer monitor. Simultaneous flow and pressure measurements were displayed on their respective consoles. Waveforms were stored on the computer disks for analysis at a later time.

After baseline measurements were obtained, a tourniquet was placed around the proximal external iliac artery until flow was reduced by 50% of the resting state; simultaneous waveforms from all three sensors were then recorded.

Linear regression analysis was used to analyze the waveforms obtained from the PGS, the pressure transducer, and the electromagnetic flow meter.

RESULTS

In Vitro Testing

Figure 1 shows the tracings obtained from the sensor in an illustrative experiment; a steady signal in the 60-80 mV range (Fig. 1a) was obtained. Upon occlusion of the outflow tract from the branch containing the graft, the signal strength increased slightly. (Fig. 1b) Occlusion of the inflow tract resulted in a markedly diminished waveform with wide pulse contour. (Fig. 1c)

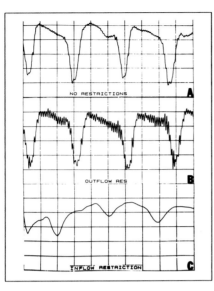

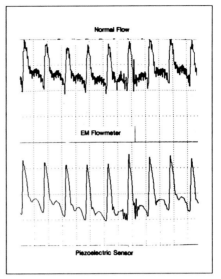

Figure 1. A. Tracing obtained from the piezoelectric sensor wrapped around a PTFE graft being perfused by a pulsatile pump at a flow rate of 300 ml/minute. A steady signal in the 60-80 mV range was obtained.
B. With occlusion of the outlfow tract from the graft, there was turbulence and a slight increase in the signal strength.
C. Occlusion of the inflow tract resulted in a markedly diminished waveform with a wide pulse contour.

Figure 2. Tracings obtained from the piezoelectric sensor placed around a PTFE graft inserted as an iliofemoral graft in a dog and the electromagnetic flowmeter placed around the common femoral artery distal to the PTFE graft.

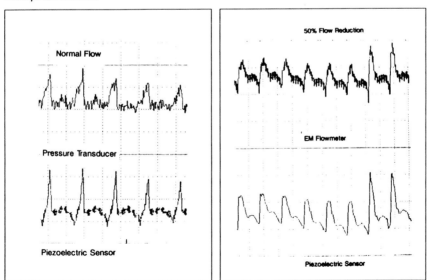

Figure 3. Tracings obtained from the piezoelectric sensor placed around a PTFE graft inserted an an iliofemoral graft in a dog and the intraluminal pressure transducer placed in PTFE graft.

Figure 4. Tracings obtained from the piezoelectric sensor and the electromagnetic flowmeter after reduction of blood flow to 50% of normal.

In vivo testing

In the resting state, the mean blood flow was 123 + 16 ml and the mean intraluminal pressure was 124/78 mm Hg. There was excellent correlation between the PVF2 sensor and flow recording (r>0.99) (Fig. 2), as well as the PVF2 sensor and the intraluminal pressure (r>0.93). (Fig. 3) Recordings comparing the three sensors were made after the tourniquet was applied. (Figs. 4 and 5) There was a remarkable similarity with a very high correlation between the three sensors, between the sensor and the flow meter (r>0.99), and the sensor and the pressure signal (r>0.92).

COMMENTS

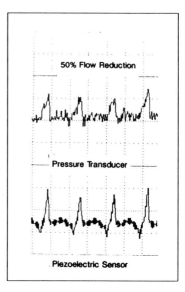

Figure 5. Tracings obtained from the piezoelectric sensor and the pressure transducer after flow reduction of blood flow to 50% of normal.

In a prospective, randomized, multicenter comparison of autologous saphenous vein (ASV) and expanded PTFE grafts in infrainguinal arterial reconstructions,[9] it was shown that the primary patency rate of ASV grafts was superior to that of PTFE grafts in femoropopliteal reconstruction. The four-year patency rates for below knee popliteal bypasses were 76% and 54% for ASV and PTFE, respectively. For infrapopliteal bypasses, the difference in the four-year patency rates was even more striking—49% for ASV compared with 12% for PTFE. This study documents the high primary failure rate of infrainguinal bypasses, particularly when PTFE grafts are anastomosed to the distal tibial or peroneal arteries.

There are multiple reasons for graft failure. Within the first month of operation, graft failure may be due to technical error, incorrect choice of operation, or transient hypotension.[10,11] Late graft failure, occurring after the first postoperative month, may be the result of anastomotic neointimal hyperplasia or the progression of atherosclerosis, or may be of undetermined etiology.[1-3,5]

Graft failure may result in the return of the patient's original symptoms, decreased or absent distal pulses, or other signs of vascular insufficiency. Noninvasive studies that detect graft failure should be followed by angiography to confirm the presence of graft thrombosis. It has been established that a number of these clinically failed grafts are actually patent, and these are referred to as "failing grafts."[12,13] If these grafts are followed closely without intervention, they will ultimately progress to graft occlusion.

It is important to detect a bypass graft when it is failing because the management and treatment of such grafts are different from those used for a failed graft. It has been shown that failing grafts can be managed with transcutaneous angioplasty of stenotic lesions in more than 70% of cases.[1,12] Reoperation is reserved for angioplastic failures or occluded arterial segments. Once a thrombosis has developed in a graft, reoperation and performance of often complex procedures are necessary to achieve limb salvage, and the operative mortality is as high as 5%.[10,11] Treatment prior to thrombosis is simpler, results in better long-term patency and limb salvage rates, and has a lower mortality rate. Graft salvage was possible in 80% of failing grafts, while only 25% of failed grafts could be effectively salvaged.[12]

At present, recognition of the failing bypass graft can be accomplished by routine follow-up with physical examination and noninvasive studies [5,7,8,14] such as pulse volume recordings, ankle systolic blood pressure, and Doppler/ ultrasound (duplex) examination. For adequate surveillance, these studies have to be performed at least every three months. The studies take at least 1 hour to complete and cost around $300. Furthermore, serial studies using ankle systolic blood pressure measurements alone failed to predict graft failure even if there was significant deterioration in the pressures.[7]

Piezoelectric polymers are widely used in science and industry. They can be easily produced in the form of an ultra-thin film that can conform to a variety of shapes. Polyvinylidene fluoride is the polymer with the strongest piezoelectric activity.[16] Applications of piezoelectric polymers include pyroelectric, electromagnetic, and mechanical to electrical transduction.[16] It is this last property—the transformation of minute mechanical deformations into electrical signals—which makes it useful for evaluating arterial bypass graft function. A study comparing PGSs to intraluminal pressure transducer to detect pressure changes in PTFE in vitro and in vivo vascular implants revealed no significant differences between the two instruments.[17] Studies correlating PGS output with actual blood flow in PTFE grafts, determined by an electromagnetic flow probe, have not been performed.

Hopefully, a PGS will prove to be more accurate than noninvasive studies in the detection of failing bypass grafts. the overall cost will be less than that of these other modalities and it will be easier to use.

REFERENCES

1. Veith FJ, Weiser RK, Gupta, SK et al. Diagnosis and Management of failing lower extremity arterial reconstructions prior to graft occlusion. J Cardiovasc Surg 1984; 25(5):381-384.
2. Ascer E, Collier P, Gupta SK, Veith FJ. Reoperation for PTFE bypass failure: The importance of distal outflow site and operative technique in determining outcome. J Vasc Surg 1987; 5:298-310.
3. Berkowitz HD, Hobbs CL, Roberts B et al. Value of routine vascular laboratory stuides to identify vein graft stenosis. Surgery 1981; 90:971-9.
4. Sanchez LA, Gupta SK, Veith FJ et al. A 10-year experience with one hundred fifty failing or threatened vein and polytetrafluorethylene arterial bypass grafts. J Vasc Surg 1991; 14:736-738.
5. Whittemore AD, Clowes, AW, Couch NP et al. Secondary femoropopliteal reconstruction. Ann Surg 1981; 193: 35-42.
6. Sladen JG, Gilmour JL. Vein graft stenosis. Am J Surg 1981; 141: 549-53.
7. Griff MJ, Nicolaides AN, Wolfe JHN. Detection and grading of femorodistal vein graft stenosis: duplex velocity measurements compared with angiography. J Vasc. Surg 1988; 8:661-6.
8. Blackshear WM, Thiele BL, Strandness DE. Natural history of above- and below-knee femoropopliteal grafts. Am J Surg 1980; 140: 234-41.

9. Barnes RW, Thompson BW, MacDonald CM et al. Serial nonivasive studies do not herald postoperative failure of femoropopliteal or femorotibial bypass grafts. Ann Surg 1989; 210: 486-94.

10. Green RM, MacNamara J, Ouriel K et al. Comparison of infrainguinal graft surveillance techniques. J Vasc Surg 1990; 11: 207-15.

11. Veith FJ, Gupta SK, Ascer E. Six year prospective multicenter randomized comparison of autologous saphenous vein and expanded polytetrafluorethylene grafts in infrainguinal arterial reconstructions. J Vasc Surg 1986; 3:104-14.

12. Veith FJ, Gupta SK, Daly V. Management of early and late thrombosis of expanded polytetraflouroethylene (PTFE) femoropopliteal bypass graft: Favorable prognosis with appropriate reoperation. Surgery 1980; 87: 581-7.

13. Veith FJ, Ascer E, Gupta SK et al. Management of the occluded and failing PTFE graft. Acta Chir Scan 1987; 538: 117-21.

14. Veith FJ, Weiser RK, Gupta SK et al. Diagnosis and management of failing lower extremity arterial reconstructions prior to graft occlusion. J Cardiovasc Surg 1984; 25: 381-4.

15. O'Mara CS, Flinn WR, Johnson ND et al. Recognition and surgical management of patent but hemodynamically failed arterial grafts. Ann Surg 1981; 193: 467-73.

16. Bandyk DF, Cato RF, Towne JB. A low-flow velocity predicts failure of femoropopliteal and femorotibial bypass grafts. Surgery 1985; 98: 799-809.

17. Kawai H. The piezoelectricity of poly (vinylident fluoride) Jap J Appl Physics 1969; 8:975-79.

18. Marcus MA. Ferroelectric polymers and their applications. Presented at the Fifth International Meeting of Ferroelectricity, Pennsylvania State University, College Park, PA August 17-21, 1981.

19. Dario P, Richardson PD, Galleti PM. Monitoring of prosthetic vascular grafts using piezoelectirc polymer sensors. Trans Am Soc Artif Intern Organs 1983; 29: 318-23.

CHAPTER 8

MANAGEMENT OF FAILING GRAFTS DETECTED DURING SURVEILLANCE

Luis A. Sanchez
Sushil K. Gupta
Frank J. Veith

Over the past 10 years, advances in vascular surgery and interventional radiology have resulted in improved primary and secondary patency rates of lower extremity bypass grafts with improved limb salvage rates.[1] However, these grafts have a steady attrition due to graft thrombosis. In the early 1980s, it was recognized that some grafts that appeared to be thrombosed with a decrease in the distal pulses, return of ischemic symptoms, or worsening noninvasive tests were still patent with diminished flow.[2-6] These hemodynamically failed arterial reconstructions have been termed "failing grafts."[4] Since then, other investigators have also described grafts in the "failing state" and noted that this condition may occur with few or no clinically evident signs or symptoms, and can only be detected through a rigorous protocol of surveillance. Early experience with failing grafts indicates that without prompt intervention, thrombosis usually occurs with return of limb-threatening ischemia. When treatment is instituted before thrombosis occurs, the management techniques are easier and can lead to improved secondary patency and limb salvage rates.[3-9]

Most of the early reports have largely described lesions with and associated with vein grafts. The failing state may occur with PTFE arterial reconstructions as well, and responsible lesions may be present in the inflow arteries, outflow arteries, within the graft or at the proximal or distal anastomosis.[4,5,12] The present report describes a 10-year experience with management of failing arterial reconstructions. The purpose of this study was to determine the frequency and etiology of lesions causing the failing state in vein and PTFE grafts and to outline a strategy for managing these graft-threatening lesions.

Reproduced from Sanchez LA, Gupta SK, Veith FJ et al. A 10-year experience with 150 failing or threatened vein and polytetrafluoroethylene arterial bypass grafts. Journal of Vascular Surgery 1991; 14:729-738, with permission from Mosby-Year Book, Inc.

MATERIALS AND METHODS

PATIENT SELECTION

During the period from January 1, 1980 to December 21, 1989, 2187 patients at the Montefiore Medical Center underwent lower extremity revascularization for limb-threatening ischemia.[1] Postoperatively, all patients received careful physical examination every two weeks for the first month, and every one to three months during the first postoperative year. During the second year, patients were examined every three months and every three to six months thereafter as long as no deterioration in their status was detected. Noninvasive examinations, including ankle brachial indices (ABIs) and pulse volume recordings (PVRs), were performed periodically and whenever graft failure was suspected by history or by a change in the physical examination. During the last five years, all patients underwent routine postoperative Doppler examination and more recently, duplex scanning at regular intervals (every 3-6 months). During the 10-year period, 125 grafts failed within one month of the arterial reconstruction and 637 grafts occluded during the follow-up period. The occluded grafts were excluded from the study. When severe hemodynamic compromise or graft occlusion was suspected, urgent arteriography was performed. All patients found to have patent grafts associated with hemodynamically significant lesions in angiography were retrospectively reviewed.

Grafts that were found to be failing within one month of the initial bypass procedure were excluded from this review. The remaining 150 grafts in 138 patients presented 226 times in the failing state. One hundred seventy-eight failing grafts (78%) resulted in recurrent symptoms which led to the diagnosis. Thirty-four (15%) were initially detected by changes in the patient's pulse status or recurrent symptoms; 8 (4%) were unsuspected and were detected during diagnostic arteriography for the contralateral lower extremity; and 6 (3%) were identified by routine noninvasive testing (duplex scanning, ABIs or both). One hundred and forty (62%) of the failing grafts presented within 12 months of the original operation; 160 (71%) within 18 months; and 178 (79%) within two years. Forty-eight (21%) presented more than two years after the original operation.

All patients in this study were followed for 4-120 months after their initial operation, with a mean follow-up of 44 months. Their ages ranged from 36 to 86 years (mean of 68 years). There were 81 males and 57 females.

Critical limb-threatening ischemia was the indication for the initial bypass procedure in all cases. Ischemic rest pain was present in 55 (37%) patients, gangrene in 45 (30%), and nonhealing ulcer in 50 (33%). The risk factors for peripheral vascular disease in this group of patients included diabetes mellitus (63%), atherosclerotic heart disease (63%), smoking (60%), hypertension (45%), myocardial infarction (42%), and symptomatic cerebrovascular disease (15%). Most patients had multiple risk factors.

DATA COLLECTION AND ANALYSIS

Data were obtained from a registry maintained on an IBM microcomputer relational database (DataEase International) which was specifically adapted for the monitoring of vascular patients.[13] Eleven (8%) of 138 patients were lost to follow-up. The data were analyzed by the cumulative life table

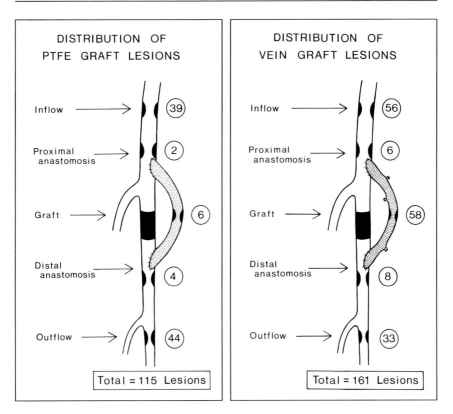

Figure 1. Distribution of 115 lesions associated with failing PTFE graft lesions

Figure 2. Distribution of lesions associated with 161 failing vein grafts

Table 1. Distribution and treatment of lesions associated with all failing grafts

	Lesions (No.)	PTA* (No.)	PTA* (%)	Surgery (No.)	Surgery (%)	Type of Operation** (No.)
Inflow	99	53	(54%)	46	(46%)	PE (46)
Graft	67	58	(87%)	9	(13%)	P/I (7) I (2)
Anastomotic	21	14	(67%)	7	33%)	PE (1) P/I (4) I (1) DE (1)
Outflow	98	31	(32%)	67	(68%)	DE (67)
TOTAL	285	156	(55%)	129	(45%)	129

*PTA=Percutaneous transluminal balloon angioplasty.
**PE=Proximal extension; PI=patch/intraluminal defect excision; I=interposition graft; DE=distal extension.

method. The secondary patency rate was calculated using the ultimate patency or the ultimate failure of the graft as the endpoint, irrespective of the intervention (percutaneous transluminal balloon angioplasty [PTA], surgery, or both) for the failing state.[14] The *extended patency* was calculated from the time of the first intervention for the failing state to the most recent endpoint. The significance of the differences between life tables was determined by the log rank sum test for comparison of life tables, and the standard error for each interval was calculated using the method of Peto et al.[16] Statistical significance was assumed at the 95% confidence level (p <.05).

RESULTS

DISTRIBUTION OF LESIONS

There were 150 grafts at risk of failure in 138 patients (7 axillofemoral; 18 femorofemoral; 5 aortofemoral; 69 femoropopliteal; 47 femorodistal; 4

Table 2. Distribution and treatment of lesions associated with PTFE grafts

	Lesions (No.)	PTA (No.)	Surgery (No.)
Inflow	39	17	22
Proximal anastomosis	2	2	0
Graft	6	4	2
Distal anastomosis	4	1	3
Outflow	64	9	55
TOTAL	115	33 (29%)	82 (71%)

Table 3. Distribution and treatment of lesions associated with vein grafts

	Lesions (No.)	PTA (No.)	Surgery (No.)
Inflow	56	33	23
Proximal anastomosis	6	4	2
Graft	58	52	6
Distal anastomosis	8	7	1
Outflow	33	22	11
TOTAL	161	118 (73%)	43 (27%)

sequential femoro-popliteal-distal grafts). A total of 285 lesions were identified. There were 99 (35%) in the inflow tract, 98 (34%) in the outflow tract, 67 (24%) within in the body of the graft, and 21 (7%) at either or both anastomotic sites. (Table 1) One hundred and fifteen lesions were associated with 74 PTFE grafts (Table 2, Fig. 1) and 161 lesions were associated with 72 vein grafts. (Table 3, Fig. 2) Four composite vein/PTFE grafts had 9 associated lesions (5 in inflow or outflow vessels; 3 within the graft; 1 at the distal anastomosis).

TREATMENT

The treatment of graft-threatening lesions included PTA, with or without thrombolytic therapy, and surgical interventions. Treatment decisions were made by the attending surgeon in consultation with an interventional radiologist. Balloon angioplasty was used for short (<5 cm) inflow lesions of the iliac, femoral and popliteal arteries, selected short (<3 cm) outflow lesions of the femoral, popliteal and tibial arteries, and some short (<5 cm) vein graft and anastomotic lesions. Surgical repair was used for long (>5 cm), multiple, or segmental occlusive lesions. Additionally, PTA failures were managed surgically.

PERCUTANEOUS BALLOON ANGIOPLASTY

A total of 156 (56%) of the 285 lesions were treated with balloon angioplasty. (Table 1) Fifty-three (54%) of 99 inflow lesions were treated by PTA. These inflow lesions included all gradient producing stenoses (both with and without papaverine injection) and all high-grade stenoses (>70% reduction in lumen diameter). Thirty-one (32%) of 98 arterial outflow lesions were treated with PTA using previously described methods.[16] Fourteen (67%) of 21 anastomotic lesions and 58 (87%) of 107 graft lesions were treated by PTA. Two grafts were managed with intraluminal thrombolytic therapy using urokinase infusion. In these two cases, following clot lysis the underlying atherosclerotic lesions were treated by PTA.

SURGERY

A total of 129 (45%) of the 285 lesions, including long (>5 cm), diffuse or occlusive lesions, lesions not accessible or amenable to balloon angioplasty, and balloon angioplasty failures, were treated surgically. (Table 1) Surgical procedures included patch graft angioplasty, valve or intramural defect excision, short interposition graft, and proximal and distal extensions. Although vein patches and vein grafts were used preferentially for all infrainguinal procedures, PTFE was used when vein was unavailable or inadequate. Surgical interventions were necessary for 46 (46%) of the 99 inflow lesions, 9 (13%) of the 67 graft lesions, 7 (33%) of the 21 anastomotic lesions, and 67 (68%) of the 98 outflow lesions. (Table 1)

FAILING PTFE GRAFTS

Surgical intervention was the principal treatment for 82 (71%) of the 115 graft-threatening lesions associated with PTFE grafts. Balloon angioplasty was used for the remaining 33 lesions. (Table 2, Fig. 3) The majority of these lesions were in the inflow or outflow arteries. Only six intraluminal defects were noted within prosthetic grafts. Two graft lesions were treated by balloon angioplasty alone and two required thrombolytic therapy in combination with balloon angioplasty. The two remaining graft lesions were excised.

Failing Vein Grafts

Seventy-three percent (118/161) of the lesions associated with vein grafts were treated with PTA. (Table 3, Fig. 4) Surgery was performed for the remaining 43 lesions, including multiple lesions, long lesions and angioplasty failures. Fifty-four (90%) of the 58 intragraft vein lesions were treated with PTA, with initial success in 52. For the purpose of evaluating the use of balloon angioplasty in the treatment of lesions within vein grafts, we divided the lesions into two groups: simple and complex. Simple lesions are vein graft lesions <1.5 cm in length within veins that are $\geq$1.5 cm in length or within grafts <3 mm in minimal diameter.

The six-year secondary patency rate for treated failing grafts was 65%. (Table 4) At five years, the extended patency rate for failing grafts was 56% and the overall six-year limb salvage rate was 75%. The six-year patient survival rate was 54%. The cumulative life table secondary patency rates for failing grafts were calculated with respect to initial treatment (PTA or surgery). The five-year secondary patency rate for failing grafts initially treated with PTA (58%) was not significantly different (p=0.25) from the patency rate for failing grafts treated initially with surgery (71%). (Table 5) In addition, there was no significant difference (p=0.25) between the secondary patency rates of failing grafts treated only with PTA (67% four-year secondary patency) and those treated only with surgery (81% four-year secondary patency). (Table 5) The secondary patency rates were also calculated with respect to the number of interventions for recurrent failing states. At four

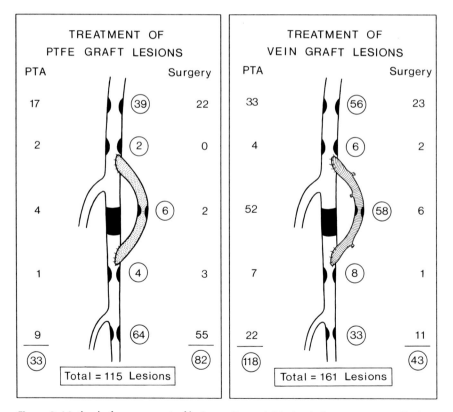

Figure 3. Method of mangement of lesions associated with failing PTFE grafts.

Figure 4. Method of management of lesions associated with failing vein graft lesions.

years, the secondary patency rates for failing grafts after a single intervention, two interventions and three or more interventions were 78%, 77% and 63% respectively. These patency rates were not significantly different (≥ 0.25). Vein grafts with simple lesions had an extended patency rate of 93% at 24 months after treatment. This was significantly better (p=0.001) than the 54% extended patency rate for vein grafts with complex lesions. The 30-day mortality rate following treatment of failing grafts was 0.7%. No mortalities were associated with PTA. Two perforations as a result of PTA required surgical repair.

DISCUSSION

A failing graft is a conduit threatened by a hemodynamically significant lesion within the graft, inflow arteries, or outflow arteries. Our early experience with 38 failing grafts suggested that most patients could be successfully treated with PTA or simple surgical procedures with good results.[4] The present study represents an extended experience and provides additional insights into the nature and optimal management of failing arterial reconstructions. This report reviews 285 lesions associated with 150 grafts. Since 78% of the patients were symptomatic at the time of presentation, the lesions detected in our series may have been more advanced than those reported by

Table 4. Cumulative six-year secondary graft patency rates of all failing grafts

Interval (mo.)	No. at risk	No. failed	No. withdrawn	Interval patency rate(%)	Cumulative patency rate(%)	Standard error
0-1	150	0	0	100	100	0.00
1-6	150	3	4	97.7	97.7	1.13
6-12	143	6	7	95.7	93.7	1.95
12-18	130	6	12	95.1	89.2	2.56
18-24	112	6	12	94.3	84.1	3.16
24-30	94	3	7	96.6	81.3	3.62
30-36	84	3	9	96.2	78.3	3.97
36-42	72	3	6	95.6	74.9	4.42
42-48	63	1	8	98.3	73.6	4.76
48-54	54	5	7	90.1	66.3	5.23
54-60	42	1	5	97.4	64.6	5.93
60-66	36	0	4	100	64.6	6.40
66-72	32	0	4	100	64.6	6.79

Table 5. Cumulative six-year secondary patency rates of all failing grafts initially treated with percutaneous transluminal angioplasty (PTA), initially treated with surgery, treated only with PTA and treated only with surgery

Interval (mo.)	No. at risk	No. failed	No. withdrawn	Interval patency rate(%)	Cumulative patency rate(%)	Standard error
Initially PTA						
0-1	71	0	0	100	100	0.00
1-6	71	0	2	100	100	0.00
6-12	69	4	4	94.0	94.0	2.70
12-18	61	3	8	94.7	89.0	3.70
18-24	50	5	4	89.5	79.8	5.00
24-30	41	3	4	92.3	73.6	5.90
30-36	34	1	6	96.7	71.2	6.50
36-42	27	1	3	96.0	68.4	7.30
42-48	23	1	3	95.3	65.3	8.00
48-54	19	2	3	88.5	57.8	8.50
54-60	14	0	2	100	57.8	10.00
60-66	12	0	0	100	57.8	10.00
66-72	12	0	0	100	57.8	10.00
Initially Surgery						
0-1	79	0	0	100	100	0.00
1-6	79	3	1	96.1	96.1	2.11
6-12	75	2	5	97.2	93.5	2.74
12-18	68	3	4	95.4	89.2	3.54
18-24	61	1	7	98.2	87.7	3.93
24-30	53	0	3	100	87.7	4.22
30-36	50	2	3	95.8	84.1	4.74
36-42	45	2	3	95.4	80.2	5.31
42-48	40	0	4	100	80.2	5.64
48-54	36	4	6	87.8	70.5	6.38
54-60	26	0	2	100	70.5	7.50
60-66	24	0	3	100	70.5	7.81
66-72	21	0	3	100	70.5	8.35
PTA Only						
0-1	53	0	0	100	100	0
1-6	53	0	3	100	100	0
6-12	50	4	3	91.7	91.7	3.7
12-18	43	3	5	92.5	84.9	5.0
18-24	35	4	4	87.8	74.6	6.3
24-30	27	0	4	100	74.6	7.2
30-36	23	1	4	95.2	71.71	7.9
36-42	18	1	3	93.9	66.7	9.0
42-48	14	0	2	100	66.7	10.0
Surgery Only						
0-1	71	0	0	100	100	0
1-6	71	2	1	97.1	97.1	1.94
6-12	68	1	4	98.4	95.6	2.41
12-18	63	3	4	95.0	90.9	3.44
18-24	56	1	8	98.0	89.2	3.91
24-30	47	0	2	100	89.2	4.27
30-36	45	2	3	95.4	85.1	4.89
36-42	40	2	3	94.8	80.7	5.60
42-48	35	0	4	100	80.7	5.99
						(p=0.25)

other authors. Based on this experience with longer follow-up, we have modified our original recommendations regarding the use of percutaneous balloon angioplasty and advocate this method only for short inflow or outflow graft-threatening arterial lesions, vein graft stenosis <1.5 cm in length, and anastomotic stenoses. Surgical interventions are used primarily for all other lesions responsible for failing grafts and for PTA failures.

Our initial observation that inflow, outflow, graft or anastomotic lesions will result in graft occlusion has been confirmed by others.[2-12,17] However, this is not universally accepted. Harris and coworkers have noted that some "low-grade" vein graft lesions do not progress or cause graft occlusion.[18]

It is important to determine whether bypass grafts are in the "failing state" because they required different management and result in better outcome than occluded grafts. Once thrombosis has occurred, complex surgical procedures with significant operative morbidity and mortality may be required.[4,20-22] Furthermore, the outcome of these secondary revascularizations is often poor even in the best of circumstances.[3,20-22] In addition, efforts to treat thrombosed grafts by initial thrombolytic therapy and secondary reconstructions of the underlying lesions have been discouraging.[22,23] In the present study, a six-year secondary patency rate of 65% was achieved for grafts treated in the failing state. This patency rate is superior to the results that can be obtained from secondary treatments for occluded grafts and approaches the primary patency rates for most initial bypass procedures. Salvage of the failing grafts in our series was achieved by using PTA as the initial treatment in 55% of all lesions and by using surgical interventions such as patch angioplasty, short graft extensions, or lesion excision in the remaining 45% of lesions.

The use of PTA in the treatment of vein graft stenoses is controversial, whereas its use in the treatment of arterial stenoses is generally accepted. Our results, however, support the use of PTA for both arterial and vein graft stenosis. Our group[4] and Berkowitz and Greenstein[7] demonstrated good results using PTA for vein graft stenoses, others have not been as enthusiastic.[6,9] More recently, Perler et al[11] and Whittemore et al.[24] have questioned the effectiveness of PTA compared to surgical interventions for the treatment of vein graft lesions. The present observations partially reconcile these conflicting opinions by showing that PTA may only be effective for short (<1.5 cm) vein graft lesions and anastomotic lesions.

Although the literature on failing grafts has emphasized the detection and treatment of lesions within failing vein grafts, in our series, hemodynamically significant lesions in the inflow and outflow tracts occur with almost equal frequency. In the present study, the 99 inflow lesions occurred with equal frequency in association with PTFE and vein grafts (34% and 35%, respectively). Although some of these lesions may have been caused by clamp injury,[5] most of these lesions were due to progression of atherosclerotic disease. Iliac and femoral lesions accounted for 81% of the inflow lesions treated. All of the lesions developed after the initial operation. Preoperative arteriography combined with intraoperative arterial pressure measurements, with and without the use of intraarterial papaverine, served to rule out hemodynamically significant inflow lesions at the time of the initial operation.

This study demonstrates that balloon angioplasty is effective in the management of stenotic inflow lesions. Surgery was reserved for diffuse or occlusive lesions and angioplasty failures. Outflow lesions were more diffuse, longer or inaccessible, as evidenced by the fact that 68% were treated with extensions to distal arteries. However, in 31 (32%) of all outflow lesions, a guidewire was passed through the graft and the lesion, and PTA of the lesion beyond the distal anastomosis was performed.

The results of this study demonstrate that PTFE grafts may be threatened by inflow and outflow lesions and still remain patent, permitting therapy before thrombosis occurs. Surprisingly, 6 intragraft lesions were also noted within PTFE grafts. The etiology of these lesions is uncertain. Most of these lesions occurred late and may represent organization and thickening of the inner fibrin lining that is deposited within low-flow prosthetic grafts.

There was a low frequency of anastomotic lesions in both PTFE and vein grafts in our series. Only 21 (7%) of the 285 lesions encountered were at the anastomotic sites. This could be due to a high incidence of graft thrombosis in grafts developing anastomotic intimal hyperplasia. Alternatively, our routine use of preoperative and postoperative aspirin and persantine may have decreased the incidence of anastomotic lesions in our patients.[25]

While anastomotic lesions were rare, lesions within vein grafts were common. The etiology of these lesions included focal and diffuse intimal hyperplasia and valve lesions as previously described.[3,7,10,16,17,26] Intrinsic pre-existing defects within venous conduits have also been observed and may account for some of the vein graft lesions that were detected.[26,27] All of these lesions can lead to graft thrombosis, but if detected early, graft thrombosis may be avoided and improved outcomes may be achieved.

Early recognition of failing grafts requires a protocol of close postoperative surveillance using clinical evaluation and serial noninvasive laboratory examinations. Controversy exists with regard to the frequency and type of noninvasive laboratory tests that should be used to follow these patients. Berkowitz and Greenstein[7] showed that the diagnosis of a failing graft could be made by ABIs or PVRs in 60% of limbs with significant lesions in asymptomatic patients. In contrast, Green et al[28] and Barnes et al[29] have reported that ABIs have low sensitivity, low specificity and great variability in predicting graft failure. In contrast, duplex examination has been found to be very reliable in predicting vein graft failure. Peak systolic velocities greater than 120 cm/sec or less than 45 cm/sec have been cited as criteria that indicate a failing vein graft.[8,27] Although we have noted peak systolic velocities less than 45 cm/sec in grafts that remained patent for several years without detectable lesions, these criteria mandate arteriography. In addition, frequent, careful physical examination by a skilled examiner led to the detection of 93% of the failing grafts in our study. However, it should be noted that some were only detectable by periodic duplex ultrasonography. It is likely however, that more failing grafts could have been recognized prior to graft thrombosis if duplex ultrasonography had been used more frequently during the earlier part of the study. We therefore believe that both routine physical examination and noninvasive tests should be used to detect failing grafts.[6,10,12,17]

Since most failing grafts (79%) were detected in the first two years, our present policy includes careful physical examination at frequent intervals by the same examiner for the first two postoperative years. Routine noninvasive vascular tests, including duplex ultrasonography, supplement the follow-up. Surveillance must continue beyond two years, since 21% of failing grafts were diagnosed between two and eight years postoperatively. These observations contradict the recommendations of others who believe that surveillance of lower extremity arterial reconstructions beyond 12-18 months is unnecessary.[30] Continued surveillance at regular intervals will allow these lesions to be detected and treated before they lead to graft thrombosis. The patient's interests will thus be best served if the surgeon accepts the responsibility of providing this surveillance indefinitely after the original arterial reconstruction.

REFERENCES

1. Veith FJ, Gupta SK, Wengerter KR et al. Changing arteriosclerotic disease patterns and management strategies in lower limb threatening ischemia. Ann Surg 1990; 212:402-14.
2. O'Mara CS, Flynn WR, Johnson ND et al. Recognition and surgical management of patent but hemodynamically failed arterial grafts. Ann Aurg 1981; 193:467-76.
3. Whittemore AD, Clowes AW, Couch NP, Mannick JA. Secondary femoropopliteal reconstruction. Ann Surg 1981; 193:35-42.
4. Veith FJ, Weiser RK, Gupta SK et al. Diagnosis and management of failing lower extremity arterial reconstructions prior to graft occlusion. J. Cardiovasc Surg 1984; 25:381-4.
5. Smith CR, Green RM, DeWeese, JA. Pseudoocclusion of femoropopliteal bypass grafts. Circulation 1983; 68(suppl II):88-93.
6. Cohen JR, Mannick, JA, Couch NP, Whittemore AD. Recognition and management of impending vein-graft failure. Arch Surg 1986; 121:758-9.
7. Berkowitz HD, Greenstein SM. Improved patency in reversed femoral infrapopliteal autogenous vein grafts by early detection and treatment of the failing graft. J Vasc Surg 1987; 5:755-61.
8. Bandyk DF, Schmidtt DD, Seabrook GR, Adams MB, Towne JB. Monitoring functional patency of in situ saphenous vein bypasses: The impact of a surveillance protocol and elective revision. J Vasc Surg 1989; 9:286-96.
9. Bandyk DF, Bergamini TM, Towne JB, Schmitt DD, Seabrook GR. Durability of vein graft revision: A comparison of secondary procedures. J Vasc Surg 1991; 13:200-10.
10. Bergamini TM, Towne JB, Bandyk DF, Seabrook GR, Schmitt DD. Experience of the eighty's with in situ saphenous vein bypass: Determinant factors of long-term patency. J Vasc Surg 1991; 13:137-49.
11. Perler BA, Osterman FA, Mitchell SE, Burdick JF, Williams GM. Balloon dilatation versus surgical revision of infrainguinal autogenous vein graft stenoses: Long-term follow-up. J Cardiovasc Surg 1990; 31:656-61.
12. Berkowitz HD, Greenstein S, Barker CF, Perloff LJ. Late failure of reversed vein bypass grafts. Ann Surg 989; 210:782-6.
13. Gupta SK, Veith FJ, White-Flores SA et al. A system of widespread applications of microcomputers to vascular surgery. J Vasc Surg 1984; 1:601-4.
14. Veith, FJ, Gupta SK, Daly VR. Femoropopliteal Bypass to the Isolated Popliteal Segment: Is Polytetrafluoroethylene Graft Acceptable? Surgery 1981;89:296-303.
15. Peto R, Mike MC, Armitage P et al. Design and analysis of randomized

trials requiring prolonged observations of each patient. Analysis and Examples. Br J Cancer 1977; 35:1-39.

16. Bakal CW, Sprayregen S, Scheinbaum K et al. Percutaneous transluminal angioplasty of the infrapopliteal arteries: Results in 53 patients. Am J Roent 1990; 154:171-74.

17. Szilagyi DE, Elliot JP, Hageman JH et al. Biologic fate of autogenous vein implants as arterial substitutes: Clinical, angiographic and histopathologic observations in femoropopliteal operations for atherosclerosis. Ann Surg 1973; 178:232-46.

18. Harris P, Moody P, Gould D. Vein graft surveillance improves patency in femoropopliteal bypass. Eur J Vasc Surg 1990; 4:117-21.

19. Veith FJ, Gupta SK, Daly V. Management of early and late thrombosis of expanded polytetrafluoroethylene (PTFE) femoropopliteal bypass grafts: Favorable prognosis with appropriate reoperation. Surgery 1980; 87:581-7.

20. Veith FJ, Gupta SK, Ascer E et al. Improved stagies for secondary operations on infrainguinal arteries. Ann Vasc Surg 1990; 3:85-93.

21. Bartlett ST, Olinde AJ, Flinn WR et al. The reoperative potential of infrainguinal bypass: Long-term limb and patient survival. J Vasc Surg 1987; 5:170-9.

22. Gardiner GA, Harrington DP, Koltun W et al. Salvage of occluded arterial bypass grafts by means of thrombolysis. J Vasc Surg 1990; 11:289-96.

23. Belkin M, Donaldson MC, Whittemore AD, Polak VF, Grassi CJ, Harrington DP, Mannick, JA. Observations on the use of thrombolytic agents for thrombotic occlusion of infrainguinal vein grafts. J Vasc Surg 1990; 11:289-96.

24. Whittemore AD, Donaldson MC, Mannick JA. Failure of balloon angioplasty in the treatment of graft vein stenosis. J Vasc Surg 1991; In Press.

25. Green RM, Roedersheimer LR, DeWeese JA. Effects of aspirin and dipyridamole on expanded polytetrafluorethylene graft patency. Surgery 1982; 92:1016-26.

26. Wengerter KR, Veith FJ, Gupta SK, Torres M, Harris P, Shanik G. Prospective randomized multicenter comparison of in situ and reversed vein infrapopliteal bypasses. J Vasc Surg 1991; 13:189-99.

27. Panetta TF, Wengerter KR, Marin ML, Goldsmith J, Gupta SK, Veith FJ. Unsuspected preexisting saphenous vein pathology: An unrecognized cause of vein bypass failure. J Vasc Surg 1992;15(1): 102-110,

28. Green RM, McNamara J, Ouriel K, DeWeese JA. Comparison of infrainguinal surveillance techniques. J Vasc Surg 1990; 11:207-15.

29. Barnes RW, Thompson BW, MacDonald CM et al. Serial noninvasive studies do not herald postoperative failure of femoropopliteal or femorotibial bypass grafts. Ann Surg 1989; 210:486-94.

30. Taylor PR, Wolfe JHN, Tyrrell MR, Mansfield AO, Nicolaides AN, Houston RE. Graft stenosis: Justification for 1 year surveillance. Br J Surg 1990; 77:1125-28.

CHAPTER 9

EPILOGUE

Sushil K. Gupta

Since the classic description of the mechanisms of vein graft failure by
Szilagyi[1] in 1973, vascular surgeons are aware that 25-30% of the grafts
implanted by them will develop lesions in the course of the graft itself or in
the inflow or the outflow tracts. The majority of these lesions occur within
the first year. It also has been shown that some of these lesions, if allowed to
progress, will cause significant reduction in flow and either cause symptoms
to return or lead to thrombosis of the grafts or both.

In the 1970s, graft failure usually meant complete thrombosis of the
graft. Patients usually presented with ischemic symptoms particularly if the
bypass had been necessary for limb salvage. During careful follow-up of these
patients, a number of vascular surgeons began to notice that some of the vein
grafts presumed to be thrombosed because of lack of pulses or return of
symptoms were in fact still patent but had significant reduction in flow
caused by a lesion in the inflow, proximal or distal anastomosis in the graft
itself or in the outflow tract.[2-4] This was termed "pseudoocclusion" or "failing
bypass graft." This phenomenon was believed to only happen with vein grafts,
since prosthetic grafts were thought to have lower thrombolytic thresholds
and could not stay patent at low flows[5] but Veith et al[4] and Sanchez et al[6] have
demonstrated that "failing graft" phenomenon can also occur with ePTFE
grafts. Recognizing a failing vein graft is very important since vein graft
thrombectomy or thrombolysis has been shown to yield poorer results and
therefore, an important conduit might be lost forever. Furthermore, all the
early reports dealing with failing grafts showed that it was much easier to fix
a short stenotic segment with patch angioplasty, short jump grafts or percutaneous transluminal angioplasty (PTA) with more predictable results than
could be achieved by grafts, thrombectomy or more complex secondary
reconstructions.

Since the clinical examination could not reliably detect these lesions and
frequent repeated angiograms were considered to be too risky and costly,
noninvasive methods were used to provide an accurate assessment of graft
function in the early and late postoperative period. The chapters by Landa,
Green, Bandyk and Buth have explored the merits and demerits of application of these methods in great detail. Clearly, color flow duplex imaging has

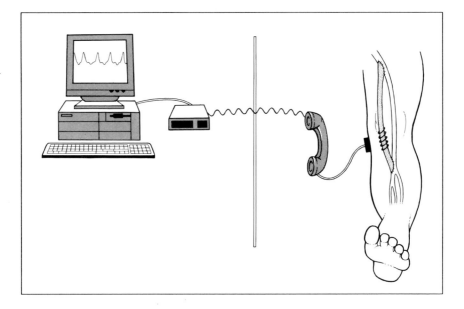

emerged as the best of these methods. This method not only has been able to detect early failing grafts but has been instrumental in elucidating the natural history of the implanted grafts.[7] Full impact of these surveillance protocols has begun to be known as more and more reports show primary assisted patency rates or secondary patency rates in the 80-90% range.[3,8]

One of the problems with surveillance that still exists is lack of uniform criteria that may direct the surgeon to intervene with confidence. Obviously, not all stenoses detected during surveillance require intervention. What stage in the evolution of stenoses constitutes impending failure beyond which the graft is irretrievably lost? Will the criteria be different for different types of grafts? A recent report by Idu et al[8] showed that when stenoses were not corrected with a diameter reduction (DR) of <50%, (using criteria outlined in Chapter 6) none thrombosed. With DR of 50-69%, four of the seven uncorrected lesions thrombosed and with DR of >70%, all three untreated grafts thrombosed. Another report by Mattos et al[9] using slightly different criteria classified graft stenoses as <50% DR and >50% DR. Ten of 38 (26%) nonrevised grafts with DR >50% occluded. However, these reports only answer some of the questions regarding discrete short lesions in the inflow or within the graft but fail to answer questions regarding long diffuse vein graft lesions or outflow lesions. A number of patients with negative scans (<50%) DR, thrombose mostly due to the outflow disease not detected by duplex scanning.

Another problem that is seen even with the most modern and rigorous surveillance studies is that a significant number of grafts (10-15%) still thrombose without a prior diagnosis of stenosis or any signs of impending problems in the interval between serial examinations. Most surveillance problems have an interval of at least three months between two consecutive examinations. Although some of these failures are a result of coagulation abnormalities, it is possible to develop lesions that go on to thrombose in this time period. It is difficult to increase the frequency of color duplex surveillance because of increased cost and inconvenience. Therefore, ultimately, the surveillance methods will have to incorporate some early warning systems that allow the graft function to be examined at a patient's home at more frequent intervals with the hope that this warning system will select the group of patients at risk so they can be monitored further with duplex scans or angiography.

With this early warning system in mind, the next question focuses on what information will provide the best indication of a failing graft. Skin temperature, blood flow; both direct or indirect and impedence of pressure all may provide clues. Obviously much work needs to be done to correlate the value of measurements done at home versus those done in a noninvasive laboratory. When the optimum mode of measurement of graft outcome is determined, a system not unlike a pacemaker monitoring system may be established. The pacemaker system allows data to be transmitted from home to a centrally located computer which can compare the output to previously stored data. A graft monitoring system could process the data and provide a warning if it does not compare favorably to predetermined criteria.

REFERENCES

1. Szilagyi DE, Elliot JP, Hageman GR et al. Biologic fate of autogenous vein implants as arterial substitutes: Clinical, angiographic and histopathologic observations in femoropopliteal operations for atherosclerosis. Ann Surg 1973; 178:232.
2. O'Mara CS, Flinn WR, Johnson ND et al. Recognition and surgical management of patent but hemodynamically failed arterial grafts. Ann Surg 1981; 193:467.
3. Smith CR, Green RM, DeWeese JA. Pseudo-occlusion of femoropopliteal bypass grafts. Circulation 1983; 68 (Suppl 11): 1188-1193.
4. Veith FJ, Weiser RK, Gupta SK et al. Diagnosis and management of failing lower extremity arterial reconstructions prior to graft occlusion. J Cardiovasc Surg 1984; 25:381.
5. Sauvage R, Walker MW, Berger K et al. Current arterial prosthesis. Experimental evaluation by implantation in the carotid and circumflex coronary arteries of the dog. Arch Surg 1979; 114:687-691.
6. Sanchez LA, Gupta SK, Veith FJ et al. A 10-year experience with 150 failing or threatened vain and polytetrafluorethylene arterial bypass grafts. J Vasc Surg 1991; 14:729-738.
7. Mills JL, Fujitani RM, Taylor SM. The characteristics and anatomic distribution of lesions that cause reversed vein grat failure: A five-year prospective study. J Vasc Surg 1993; 24:195-206.
8. Idu MM, Blankenstein JD, de Gier P et al. Impact of a color-flow duplex surveillance program on infrainguinal vein graft patency: A five-year experience. J Vasc Surg 1993; 17:42-53.
9. Mattos MA, van Bemmelen PS, Hodgson KJ et al. Does correction of stenoses identified with color duplex scanning improve infrainguinal graft patency? J Vasc Surg 1993; 17:54-66.

INDEX

Items in italics denote figures (f) or tables (t).

A

Ahn SS, 3
Angiography
  infrainguinal graft monitoring, 15, 20-22, 26, *29f*, 57-58
    intraoperative technique, 16
    intravenous digital subtraction (IV-DSA), 68
Angioplasty, 82, 89, 90, *92t*, 93-95
Angiopump®, 17
Angioscopy, 15
  infrainguinal graft monitoring, 15, 22-26, *27f*, 28, *29f*, 30
    intraoperative technique and equipment, 16-20
Ankle brachial systolic pressure index (ABI), 34-36, 44, 48, 50-53, 55, 61, 69-70
Ascer E, 14
Aspirin, 94
Atherosclerosis, 4
  graft failure, 7, 57, 68, 93

B

Bandyk DF, 51, 52, 74, 75
Barnes RW, 51, 55, 61, 94
Belkin M, 58
Berkowitz HD, 71, 93, 94
Buth J, 56

C

Creech O, 13

D

Dacron graft
  velocity waveform analysis, 37
Donaldson MC, 3, 6
Doppler ultrasound, 14. See also Velocity waveform analysis.
Duplex scanning, 37-38, *39f*
  infrainguinal graft monitoring, 49, 57-61, 61-65, 71, *72f, 72t, 73t,*74, 75, 94
    results, 65
    stenosis, 64-65
    technique, 63-64

E

Eldrup-Jorgensen J, 3
Electromagnetic flowmeter (EMF), 14
Epidermal growth factor (EGF), 5

F

Failing bypass graft. See Pseudoocclusion.
Femoropopliteal bypass
  greater saphenous vein (GSV), 1
  polytetrafluoroethylene (PTFE), 1
Fibroblast growth factor (FGF), 5
Flow patterns, *59t*

G

Gene transfection, 5
Graft failure
  early, 2-3
  hypotension, 8
  late, 3-5, 7
  mechanisms, 2, 56-57
  polytetrafluorethylene (PTFE), 89, *90f*
  sepsis, 8
  stenosis, 61-62
    ankle brachial pressure index, 69-70
    peak systolic velocity (PSV), 71, 74
  vein, 90-91
Graft revision, 74-75, 89-91, *91t, 92t,* 93-95
Graft surveillance, 55-56, 85-86
  duplex scanning, 57-61
  infrainguinal, 61-65
  polytetrafluoroethylene (PTFE), *88t*
    vein, *88t*
Greater saphenous vein (GSV) graft, 1
  in situ, 19, 23, 38
  nonreversed, 19, 23
  preparation, 2-3
  reversed, 20, 23
  selection, 2
Green RM, 79, 94
Greenstein SM, 93, 94
Griffin L, 13
Grigg MJ, 55, 74

H

Hallett JW, 3
Harris P, 93
Hemodialysis, 3
Heparin, 3
Hypercoaguable states, 3
Hypotension
  graft failure, 8

I

Idu MM, 98
Infrainguinal graft, 12-13, 68-69
  composite vein, 25
  failure
    early, 2-3
    late, 3-5
    mechanisms, 2, 56-57, 82-83
    polytetrafluorethylene (PTFE),
      89, *90f*
    vein, 90-91
  monitoring, 13, 44, 50-53, 61-65
    angiography, 15, 20-22, 26,
      29f, 57-58, 70-71
      intraoperative technique, 16
      intravenous digital subtraction
    angiography (IV-DSA), 68
    ankle brachial pressure index
      (ABI), 44, 48, 50-53, 69-70
    direct (anatomic), 15
    duplex scanning, 49, 51-52,
      58-65, 71, *72f, 72t, 73t,* 74, 75
    indirect (physiologic), 13-15
    polytetrafluoroethylene (PTFE), *88t*
    vein, *88t*
  patency, *47t*
  revision, 74-75, 89-91, *91t, 92t,*
    93-95
  stenosis, 64-65
In situ hybridization, 5
Interleukin
  -1 (IL-1), 5
  -6 (IL-6), 5
Intimal hyperplasia, 3-5
  vein graft, 5-6, 56-57, 68, 94
Intraoperative flow measurements, 14

J

Jager KA, 74

L

Laborde AL, 69, 71
Low graft velocity state, 61-62
Lupus antiphospholipid antibody, 3

M

Mattos MA, 56, 98
Mills JL, 5
Moody AP, 55
Moody P, 69, 70, 75

O

O'Donnell T, 13, 51

P

Peak systolic [flow] velocity, (PSFV or
  PSV), 4557, *58t*
  graft stenosis, 71, 74
Percutaneous transluminal angioplasty
  (PTA). See Angioplasty.
Perler BA, 93
Peroneal artery
  infrainguinal graft, 64
Persantine, 94
Piezoelectric pulse sensor, 40, *41f,* 42,
  79-80
  in vitro testing, 80, *81f,*
  in vivo testing, 80, *81f,* 82
Platelet-derived growth factor (PDGF),
  5
Plethysmography, 13
Polytetrafluoroethylene (PTFE), 1
  graft revision, *91t, 92t,* 93-95
  infrainguinal, 6-7, 69
  monitoring, *88t,* 89
  piezoelectric pulse sensor, 80-83
  velocity waveform analysis, 36, 37
Polyvinylidine fluoride, 40, 79, 83
Protein C, 3
Protein S, 3
Pseudoocclusion, 97

R

Reifsnyder R, 8

S

Sanchez LA, 68, 97
Sepsis
  graft failure, 8
Smooth muscle cells, 4
  mitogens, 5
Stirnemann P, 14
Szilagyi DE, 5, 8, 70, 97

T

Taylor PR, 69
Thrombocytopenia, 3
Thrombolytic therapy, 89
Thrombosis, 56, 57
Transcutaneous oxygen tension
   (TcPO₂), 15
Turnipseed WD, 70

U

Umbilical vein grafts, 1-2
   velocity waveform analysis, 36
Urokinase, 89

V

Valve cusp fibrosis, 69
Valvutome, 23-24
Valvulotomy, *27f*
Vein grafts
   arm, 24
   primary intraluminal pathology, 24
   stenosis, 56
Veith FJ, 97
Velocity waveform analysis, 36-37
   technique, 37

W

Whittemore AD, 93
Wolfe JHN, 70, 71